"I have been blessed in my life to be surrounded by men and women who exude bravery. My Mom and Dad, my wife Ruvé, Buck Compton from *Band of Brothers*, and now Kelsi Sheren. This incredible book is about her gut-wrenching, emotional, and heroic time spent serving the country that she loves so much. Not often when you read a book do you start from the beginning, keep reading all the way to the end, and cry for more. This book is one of them. Ruvé and I are honored not just to know that we were chosen to help Kelsi tell her story on screen, but that we were chosen by God to be her friend. It is an honor to say the least. I'm so proud of what she has done as we all should be. I cannot wait to take the story to the screen so everyone can see it in person. It is a journey of sheer triumph. I know you will agree."

—**Neal McDonough**, HBO's *Band of Brothers*

"Kelsi is an inspiration to every little girl out there wondering if they can do it or not. Kelsi shows you there are no excuses or barriers and if you want it, go and get it. Her openness about her struggles should be read by men and women alike. Her work within our community is incredible and shows everyone what is possible. Just read the book!"

—**Dean Stott**, Double World Record Breaker, UK Special Forces, and TV Presenter

"An absolutely intriguing and compelling story of a journey throughout the many trials of womanhood and what it is to be a woman in a man's world. With each new hurdle she teaches herself new methods of coping and in a fascinating way, brings to life that little voice we all have in our head. Kelsi's story is one of determination, drive, and inspiration. She may be small but she is mighty!"

—**Alana Stott**, MBE, Author, CEO, and Producer

"Bravo Zulu on your book and the honesty and resiliency you have displayed throughout your life. You are a natural fighter whose path in life forced you to face the horrors of war at a young age. This was often done with courage and determination and for that you have my upmost respect. Soldiers who have faced combat are often brought to a dark place where tears, pain, and feelings of helplessness become a way of life. While no stranger to this, you were able to eventually overcome your demons while at the same time offer support to your brothers and sisters in arms as well as their families. I wish you great success as you continue your next chapter of life and advocate for those who are still dealing with their own demons."

—**Capt. Marc Leblond**, RCA

"War isn't what Hollywood shows you. It isn't a personal triumph story where every soldier gets to overcome the enemy in a 'dark night of the soul' moment, kill the most people, return home to a parade, and live happily ever after. Most of what you've seen or read about war is a fictionalized truth. Whether it's intentional or unintentional, people in search of meaning will inevitably follow this storied path to find their own sense of connection, meaning, and truth.

"I had the fortunate opportunity to meet Kelsi during the development of this book. After reading the initial draft along with fellow combat veterans, we came to the same conclusion: She didn't represent herself to be anything she wasn't. She did her very best to honor those alongside her. She grew through the cruel pain of war. She continues to help others.

"Now, don't get me wrong. Kelsi is no angel. She's one hundred lbs of spitfire with the energetic knob turned to eleven, then snapped off. Wildly imperfect—just like everyone on this planet. We all have a path. We all make mistakes. We all have the opportunity to get our shit together and carve a positive path in this world. I hope this book serves as an example of what you can do if you take the pain shoveled upon by life, then form it into beauty."

—**Griff**, HMFIC, Combat Flip Flops, and Ranger <2>

"A true to fact illustration of the hidden injuries of war. Showing through personal experience that the issues of friendship, love, business, and war surprise the ultimate solution and that battle buddies aren't just for battle."

—**Chris Watson**, Royal Army Medical Corps and formally Black Watch 3 Scots

"Kelsi's vulnerability in sharing her personal journey brought me to tears. By personifying PTSD and the voice of self-doubt, it made me relive my experiences while in combat and transported me back to Afghanistan; Kelsi's story forced me to confront my personal baggage from the war and grow as a person."

—**Nicholas Ige**, Ranger <2>

"If this book was a selection candidate, it would pass."

—**Marcus Capone**, Founder, VETS, Inc., and former Navy SEAL

"Courage comes in all shapes and sizes. Many assume the hardest battles are fought in war. In my experience it is the battles you face after that can be the most challenging. This book captures them both."

—**Andy Stumpf**, former Navy SEAL and Host of the Podcast *Cleared Hot*

"Kelsi Sheren is a veteran voice worth listening to. Too often war stories stop after the point of action and don't invite the reader to feel the impacts of these experiences on the lives of veterans at home. Kelsi fearlessly lays out her own vulnerabilities throughout this book while also providing a captivating story along the way. For veterans, I hope this book shows that there are paths toward healing and enriching lives post-military. For everyone else, I hope this story helps bring understanding but also the universality of perseverance through trauma."

—**Jesse Gould**, former Army Ranger and Founder of Heroic Hearts Project

"An honest, raw account of combat and the hard cold realities of being a female serving on the modern battlefield. Her prose gives an inside look at not only war itself, but the war of one's self and the true cost of combat on the human mind."

—**Brian Bishop**, OIF/OEF Veteran and Host of the *Lone Element Podcast*

"Having been on deployment with Kelsi, this book took me right back to those battles that I had locked away in the far corners of my mind. She was courageous on the battlefield, moving straight toward the gunfire without hesitation, and she is a beacon of light now, fighting for those who bear the mental scars of war."

—**Daniel Venter**, Royal Artillery (FISTer)

"This book immerses the reader into the high-tempo, fast-paced operations encountered by the military in Afghanistan from the author's perspective on and off the battlefield, with the biggest battle of all so many face when they come home—the struggle of posttraumatic stress disorder from the despair and chaos to the small triumphs against this hidden killer. No matter the battle, you're never out of the fight. No one gets left behind."

—**Craig Hardie**, Combat Medic and 3 Scots Battlegroup

"Truth is in the eye of the beholder and that truth can be overwhelmingly exhilarating and powerful. Kelsi's truth took her into the darkest of places and spat her out the other side. In 2009 when Mouth—Kelsi—joined my Platoon, she was smaller than her Bergan yet heard from afar. A fucking nightmare to control but a warrior under fire and completely resolute in adversity. Her bravery under fire, physically in Afghan and mentally within herself, is inspirational. This book proves that. Grab a tissue, sit up straight, hold on, and prepare for a gut-wrenching truth from the battlefields of Afghanistan and from deep with Kelsi's soul!"

—**Stevie**, Pl Sgt, 3 SCOTS Battlegroup

"The collapse of the Afghan government was a turning point in our lives. Suddenly, like millions of Afghans, we lost everything behind. What was happening next? No one could expect different than fear, suppression, and worry. I was thinking of my family, particularly my wife, who worked for women's empowerment and had no safe hiding place. Finally, Kelsi, an angel, came for our help; she tirelessly worked to ensure my family safely evacuated Afghanistan. At one time, while I was so stressed, she messaged me, 'I'm never leaving u behind' and finally, she completed her promise. It is so merciful to have my wife and son living with me in a secure environment with equal rights and freedom."

—Enayat Nasir

"No soldier can be fully prepared for the reality of combat. Training helps, with units spending more time preparing for a deployment than they do 'on the ground.' Camaraderie and 'brotherhood' are also vital: knowing who you will be fighting alongside as well you know yourself. And knowing that you will kill and die for each other. Kelsi was not afforded either of these things. Thrown into a role that she had not been trained for, and assigned to a unit from the other side of the Atlantic Ocean, Kelsi had to hit the ground running, and Afghanistan is not a forgiving time or place. Particularly in the summer of 2009.

"Like many others, Kelsi didn't come through the experience without scars, but she has turned her pain into fuel to help others. This is one of the most unique stories to emerge from the war, and serves as a reminder that all soldiers—no matter their trade—should be ready for anything."

—**Geraint Jones**, Author and Veteran

BRASS & UNITY

ONE WOMAN'S JOURNEY THROUGH
the HELL of AFGHANISTAN and BACK

KELSI SHEREN

A KNOX PRESS BOOK
An Imprint of Permuted Press

Brass & Unity:
One Woman's Journey Through the Hell of Afghanistan and Back
© 2023 by Kelsi Sheren
All Rights Reserved

ISBN: 978-1-63758-891-8
ISBN (eBook): 978-1-63758-892-5

Cover art by Conroy Accord
Cover photo by Krupto Strategic
Section drawings by Vanessa Sheren
Interior design and composition by Greg Johnson, Textbook Perfect

Names in this book have been changed to protect the identities of those who wish to stay anonymous. This book has been written with consults from members of the British, American, and Canadian armed forces, with the best recollection of all events. Written with respect, care, and kindness.

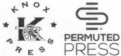

Permuted Press, LLC
New York • Nashville
permutedpress.com

Published in the United States of America
1 2 3 4 5 6 7 8 9 10

To those with whom I've served in the darkest times so that others may live. I'm grateful for you all.

To my partner in all things and better half, Roo—without you none of this would be possible. To our beautiful curly-headed explorer of all things dirty and sticky. I'm forever grateful for you bringing me into the light and showing me what it truly means to live and love.

Until Valhalla.

To the people whom I've met and worked with on this project over time: I'm grateful to you for your patience, kindness, empathy, and understanding. I am aware that, over the past four years, this hasn't been an easy process of which to be a part of, and those who have stuck it out have helped me to achieve a dream of becoming an author and helping my community. I'll never stop holding space for you in my heart. I hope you all know who you are.

To Neal and Ruvé McDonough: You'll never fully understand the love I feel for you and your family. Your big, beautiful family has welcomed me with open arms from the moment we met at our first Fire Career Rep 24-hour row-a-thon. You've continued to move mountains for me, and our next chapter together will be bigger and brighter. I thank you for taking a chance on me the way you both have.

Tali, you stood by with patience and kindness and helped me walk through the last four years of this process. I am grateful to you for this.

My parents and family, this goes without saying. I love you and thank you for the patience and grace you've given me throughout this journey to heal.

To the soldiers I served alongside, those of you I keep in contact with—Canadian, American, British, and Australian: I love you deeply, I'll never forget anything you've ever done for me. You all know who you are, some of you are mentioned in this book and others have had your name changed to protect your identity. Thank you guys so, so much.

Dr. Greg Passey, there are not enough words or pages in this world to thank you enough for the man you are, and more importantly, the doctor you are. Your integrity as a doctor is unlike anything I've ever seen or heard of. You save lives daily. You deal with the Department of Veterans Affairs' BS like a champion and have kept me moving and growing and answered the phone no matter the time. You, sir, are one of the greatest gifts the military has ever seen, and to any person who has the chance to be your patient. Thank you now and thank you later, because I know you're my doctor for life. I owe you, sir.

Jack, my son. One day you'll be old enough to read this and talk to me about it; I promise to be open and honest with you about everything and answer any questions you have. I love you, my son, you are the greatest gift and the BEST thing I've ever done in my lifetime. Thank you for choosing me as your mother; I only hope I can make you proud one day. I love you.

To my unwavering, strong, brilliant husband. I owe this all to you and your compassion, your patience, and your belief that I could do anything I wanted in this world. You really have made me believe I can achieve it all, and now I plan to because of you. Your strength is the reason I still stand today, I love you forever and always, Roo.

Contents

Foreword xiii
Author's Note xv

Prologue: Numb 1

PART 1: BRASS

Chapter One: The Start, the French 5

Chapter Two: Training 19

Chapter Three: Weapons Handling 29

Chapter Four: Posted 40

Chapter Five: Sink or Swim 54

Chapter Six: Home, Sweet Home 61

Chapter Seven: Afghanistan 66

Chapter Eight: FOB Ramrod 71

Chapter Nine: Invisible Enemy 80

Chapter Ten: "Borrowed" 86

Chapter Eleven: The Op 93

Chapter Twelve: Post Op 134

PART 2: UNITY

Chapter Thirteen: All the Meds. 145

Chapter Fourteen: Cracked. 153

Chapter Fifteen: Released 161

Chapter Sixteen: Civilian 167

Chapter Seventeen: Roo. 177

Chapter Eighteen: Restart 184

Chapter Nineteen: An Invisible Injury 191

Chapter Twenty: Stuck. 198

Chapter Twenty-One: The Beginning 208

Chapter Twenty-Two: Finding Meaning. 216

Chapter Twenty-Three: Stress, Stress, Stress 223

Chapter Twenty-Four: The New People 229

Chapter Twenty-Five: A New Chapter 240

Chapter Twenty-Six: Healing. 249

Chapter Twenty-Seven: Closure 258

Postscript: About the Veteran Crisis 279

Appendix: Coping Tips 281

Acknowledgments. 285

Foreword

Courage has many meanings for many people. For our serving military personnel and my fellow Veterans, it took courage to join the military. It takes courage to leave our loved ones behind, to miss birthdays, special occasions, holidays, and sometimes the birth of our children while serving our country in the pursuit of our foundational beliefs. It takes courage to serve overseas, to deal with war, the loss of our comrades, and then to return home to struggle with our injuries, wounds, losses, and memories. It especially takes courage to battle out of the darkness and stigma that Posttraumatic Stress Disorder (PTSD) casts on every aspect of a person's life. Kelsi has done all that her country and fellow Veterans have asked of her and so much more. Many have lost their way upon their return home and have succumbed to suicide; she managed to persevere.

Kelsi's story has taken courage to survive but even more so to tell. She has detailed the day and night struggles that she and everyone suffering from PTSD (no matter what the cause) must endure in order to survive. She has given a dark voice to the terrible brain injury that is called PTSD. It is a story of courage, strength, honor, pain, distrust, and trust, coupled with unbreakable military bonds that last a lifetime. It is a powerful and emotional story of not only surviving the dark morass of PTSD but also clawing her way out of that black hole to actually be able to live again, to be able to feel happiness, to love, to establish new friendships, a cherished family, and a life with meaning.

We lose Veterans to suicide every day—many of whom are never recognized as casualties of their military service. These are our Unknown Fallen. It has been my distinct honor to share my time, expertise, and experiences with Kelsi since 2011. Her book is an absolute must read for anyone trying to understand PTSD, cope with it, or whom want to try to make a difference and perhaps prevent more unnecessary suicides.

—*Dr. Greg Passey*
  BSc, MD, CD1, FRCPC
  Psychiatrist
  LCdr (retired)

Author's Note

This book is for my friends and fellow veterans who've lost their lives to PTS and for all of those vets who served overseas and did not fully come back. I've written this book to try to shed some light on the battle that I still fight today with PTS, in the hopes that my story might help save a life.

This book is also intended to educate those who might not understand what it's like to be a soldier and what we endure during a deployment. I want you to know what we see when we're over there and how we feel when we get home.

The truth is, all combat soldiers leave a part of themselves—or all of themselves—in a place where the dirt cuts like razors, the water doesn't flow freely, animals run wild, and the next step we take might be our last.

I want regular civilians to understand what it's like to suffer from PTSD so that they might relate to someone who is currently in the throes of it. Our veteran and first responder communities are suffering every single day with PTSD, and I want average people to know what it's like for us, not being able to go out into the general public due to this crippling disorder.

This book has been difficult to write. I was forced to think for way too long about the events that caused my PTSD and the friends I've lost, and I've been triggered a lot. But that's the thing about

PTSD. It doesn't go away; you just have to learn how to live with it. I truly hope this book will be a learning tool or a resource, or maybe a coaster on a bedside table; but as long as it helps even one person, it will all be worth it.

I never thought there would be a day in my life when I would be able to say something like that. I didn't think I'd make it to this point in healing myself, let alone trying to help others who are suffering, too. I'm sick and tired of my friends dying by suicide, overseas and at home. They're fighting in a war that is killing on both sides, physically and mentally affecting generations to come.

The contents of this book are uncomfortable. There are some very graphic details that may not be suitable for those under the age of sixteen or anyone with a weak stomach. But these things are the reality of war, and they were my reality.

War doesn't leave you when you come home.

Please let my story be one of hope, perseverance, and persistence, because we cannot lose any more people to this mental health crisis in our veteran and first responder communities. Please reach out to anyone you know who is struggling. Reach out and give a hand, even if that means pushing someone when he or she might not recognize the signs alone. You could be the thing, the person, the hope that saves someone's life.

If you need immediate assistance, call the Veteran Crisis Hotline at 1-800-273-8255 and press 1.

Chat online, or send a text to 838255 to receive confidential support twenty-four hours a day, seven days a week, 365 days a year.

USA: The 988 Suicide & Crisis Lifeline is a national network of local crisis centers that provides free and confidential emotional support to people in suicidal crisis or emotional distress 24 hours a day, 7 days a week in the United States.

I'M PTSD: LET ME INTRODUCE MYSELF

I've been called by different names over the years: Combat fatigue. Exhaustion. Soldier's heart. Shell shock. Post-Vietnam syndrome.

Most know me now as PTSD.

I don't care what you call me.

When I take you, you're *mine*.

I've claimed the lives of Spartans and countless so-called gladiators.

I take good guys, bad guys, the young and the old, and I like the *strongest* ones most of all because I prefer a challenge.

I've been *killing* for as long as wars have been waged. Since the advent of time.

My method is simple. I mess with your *head* until you can't take it anymore.

You learn to *live* with me, or you won't.

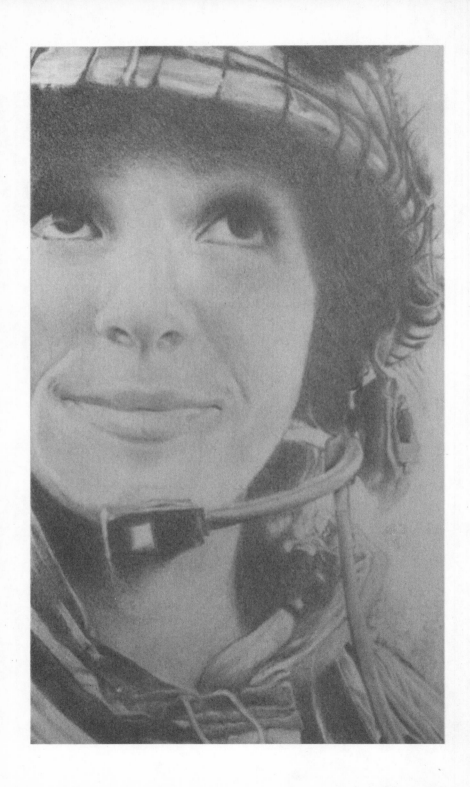

PROLOGUE

Numb

Panjwai District, Afghanistan, 0100 Hours, June 2009

I step off the Chinook onto a hot, dark landing zone with three units of the British military.

My legs are numb, as if someone was sitting on them for the entire flight. The gate opens. Everyone pushes out from the hold, and I collapse on the metal lift, which is basically at the edge of safety and Hell.

My chest tightens, and my fingers clench onto the helicopter. My feet won't move, and my world goes black as I slip in and out of consciousness. Hot air from the chopper blades presses down on me, and then someone's hand digs into my back. He leans down and screams in my ear in a thick Scottish accent, "AYE MOVE, LET'S GO!"

He lifts my whole body off the cold floor of the Chinook and pushes me out onto the Panjwai ground. The night sky keeps the heat at bay for now—almost beautiful. There is nothing, absolutely nothing, impeding the glow of the stars. It is strangely peaceful and serene, although it's one of the most dangerous places for NATO forces to be in Afghanistan—home of the Taliban. I hear nothing and everything all at once, yet this silence only lasts a moment. The quiet evening turns to war with the roar of the Chinook's blades cutting through the air.

We march onward to God knows where. My heart beats so fast in my chest, and so loud, I feel as if everyone can hear it, even with all the boots crunching on the ground.

There's no time to stand still; the feeling rushes back into my legs like a shot of adrenaline to the heart. As I begin to run, I quickly realize how uneven and hard the ground is and that it's likely littered with improvised explosive devices (IEDs).

The dry grass whips around like we're in the middle of a twister, the Chinook tossing rocks, dirt, and sand as it gets into a new position. I pull my scarf up over my face to shield my nose and mouth from flying debris.

One of the sergeants screams, "Stay with the dog handler! Just follow him, and you'll be fine!"

Before we left for this week-long op, I was told, "We don't use female searchers, really, so we probably won't need you much."

Famous last words.

PART 1

BRASS

ONE

The Start, the French

January 3, 2008

The drive with my parents from our home in Campbellford, Ontario, to the Canadian Forces Leadership and Recruit School and military base in St. Jean-sur-Richelieu, on the outskirts of Quebec, is a grueling five-hour trip. Mostly it is silent, each of us lost in our own thoughts. In the rear-view mirror, Dad's eyes watch me. They are softer than usual, and his furrowed brow doesn't lift during the entire trip.

Sprawled across the back seat, all five feet and 104 pounds of me, my eighteen-year-old self, ready, willing, and, I hope, able to become a soldier and deploy to parts unknown, I have a flashback. I can see myself at age twelve, braces on my teeth, in Tae Kwon Do class.

"Kelsi, shortstop," one of the girls shouts into my face.

I press my hands against my ears, and her words are muffled. Their mouths still move, and I can see their angry grins and arms cheering wildly. I can also see myself in the dojo's large mirrors. I am flat as a board and my hair is cut short. I cut it to be more agile on the mat; when I'm not training, I place large headphones over my cropped hair and listen to Eminem spit vitriol as I plan my next fight.

I look down from the mirror, trying not to face any of the images confronting me.

Hands slam against my shoulders, pushing me toward a group circling around me. I stumble forward to a raw cry of "Tinsel Teeth!" in unison. A shove in the other direction. "Tin Grin." I step back, but the pushing doesn't stop. My legs give way, but I stand up straight and run toward the crowd. One boy lunges forward. "You're too weak, zipper lips," and he rips off my beloved tear-away pants.

I clench my fists. This is what my long hours on the Tae Kwon Do mats are for. To move quickly. To bring down an opponent twice my size. I strike with one fist, and as his body flies backward, the group steps away from me. I walk away so they don't see my tears, biting my lip so hard my braces cut my skin. I didn't train to fight bullies. I'm better than that. But if I have to—so be it. I can show any doubters that I'm not as small and weak as I look.

Six years later, the Army recruiter who accepted my application wanted to know why a "shortstop" like me was so eager to put myself in harm's way. Of course I told him that I wanted to serve my country. There was another part of me, however, that knew I was still that same little girl fighting in Tae Kwon Do class, eager to prove that despite my appearance, I was strong—a perfect candidate for the Army.

Now I am on my way to make good on both of those promises. I lean against the car window, enough to see my mom's profile as she stares at the passing scenery. For a moment, her strong jaw line quivers and her words from last night replay in my mind: "I always suspected you might join the military one day." Whether or not she agrees with the decision, I'll never know, but that's Mom. She has always been my rock. She sacrificed everything and gave up her job to stay home when my brother and I were kids. How many times did I call home crying because someone was bullying me or because I forgot to bring a lunch to school? No matter what she was doing, she would drop everything for Dillon and I. How did she do all of that and still manage to put dinner on the table every night? My parents have made us their entire life, and now I'm going to be so far away.

For the first month of my training, I won't even be able to call my parents. I've never been out of touch with them for such a long period, even with Dad being a long-haul trucker for my entire childhood. No matter how far away he was, he called us from the road almost every night to see what we were up to, and he was home as often as he could be.

We park outside a big concrete institutional building with tiny windows, the place where I'll be living for the next few weeks. When we get out of the car, the wind smacks me in the face, my eyes water, and my nose starts to run. Mom's long blonde hair tosses around her head, and the wind grabs the long gray whiskers on Dad's chin and lifts the ball cap off his balding head. Somehow, they look older, wearier, but they are by my side, stone-faced and strong, here for me now like they've always been.

We all look at the soldiers running around the building. Some of them are in green uniforms and boots, others are in shorts, sweaters, toques, and sneakers. While some look happy, others look like they might collapse. None of them look at me.

I turn back toward my parents as I shield my eyes from the sun. Mom opens and closes her mouth, but no words come out. We can see our breath, and the air smells like snow.

They aren't allowed past this point, so I give Mom a hug; and when she lets go, wiping her tears, Dad puts his arms around me. With his beard on my cheek, his voice cracks as he manages his usual farewell. "See ya, kid. Love ya." He's said these words to me many times before leaving in his big rig.

I don't show them how nervous I am, because I don't want them to worry about me being away any more than they have to. They head back to the car, leaving me with a rugby bag that's bigger than I am, which, at my size, doesn't take much.

Heaving the bag up over my shoulder, I enter the building where shouts and loud footsteps echo in the hallway. Young men in starched and pressed uniforms march past me, swinging stiff arms, facing forward with stern expressions, and pressing syncopated boot heels into the floor.

What the hell did I sign up for?

After a few minutes, I figure out where I'm supposed to be, and a big, solid-looking man pulls me into a classroom. I soon learn he's a sergeant. He tells me, "Put down your bag, find the envelope with your name on it, then sit down and shut up."

"Yes, sir."

"What did you call me?" he barks as he leans into my flushed face. Now I know rule number one: Never, ever, call a sergeant "sir." The other members of my troop pile into the classroom. Their shoes squeak on the floor, and they're all frantically trying to find their names on the envelopes so the sergeant doesn't yell at them. His voice booms over the chaos: "Read everything inside the envelope, sign where indicated, and then climb the nine flights of stairs with your bags, up to your pod, and do it fast."

I now consider throwing out my bag. Rule number two: Pack lightly. We race upstairs as quickly as we can and start to settle into the crammed dorm-like place, and through sheer luck, I have a small room to myself.

My troop is mostly guys, with maybe six women. I try to make small talk with them, but none of them seem interested in chatting. Either they're as nervous as I am, or they're not interested in befriending me.

Some people go to bed right away while others unpack. I choose to finish the homework in the envelope because I don't want to piss off the red-faced sergeant.

The instructions are: *In a few pages, describe why you joined the military, what made you decide on the trade you chose, and a little bit about yourself.*

Snow pelts against the window, and I stare into the dark evening before I start writing, remembering the moment that prompted me to join the Army.

My name is Kelsi Burns. I joined the Army because I want to prove to all of the assholes from my small town that I am not weak just because I'm small. I am joining the Army because I'm looking for a place to belong, where my physical abilities will count for something. Because I want to help people. Because I don't know what else I can do after my coach ruined my plans for the future by making a stupid decision that broke my trust and shattered my dreams—

I tear the paper out and crumple it up. I have to sound tough, like a soldier would, so I start again.

My name is Kelsi Burns. I'm eighteen years old, and my parents are truck drivers who live in Campbellford, Ontario. My brother Dillon and I used to drive cross-country in the cab with my dad. I loved seeing Canada, and I loved traveling. I always knew there was more out there for me than Campbellford, and joining the Army, to me, equals freedom and a chance to see the world.

I was bullied the whole time I was in school, both physically and verbally. I don't know a time when I wasn't bullied for something. People pushed me around and told me I was weak. I've always felt the need to fight and prove myself tougher than everyone else, because I'm small. I was told I couldn't do things because of my size, so I always tried my best to prove that I could. My parents always pushed me to work hard, and they made me believe I can do anything I want if I put in the effort. I'm thankful they made me so strong.

When I was four years old, my mother signed me up for Tae Kwon Do, and I fell in love with it. I lived and breathed it, trained and fought competitively for eight years—I even taught classes. I earned my black belt when I was eleven years old. I learned who I was on those mats. I found determination and spirit and passion, and I planned to be a professional athlete. When I found out that my coach made a very stupid decision that jeopardized my training and hurt a lot of people, I was angry for a long time. I lost my ability to trust, and I lost my future thanks to his poor decision.

Without Tae Kwon Do, I found it hard to get through high school. My friend Lisa Gawley introduced me to rugby, which was a great way to get out anger. Rugby was filling my time, but it wasn't making me happy. I couldn't wait to get out of high school and to leave Campbellford. I went to college in Ottawa just to get away. I was accepted into a travel and tourism program that I didn't care about, and I was struggling, feeling like I had no purpose.

On Remembrance Day last November, I went to a service in Ottawa, and on my way home, I chatted with an older female veteran on the bus. I can't explain why, but I felt like I was supposed to meet her. She told me about her experience being a pilot in the Air Force, and I thought she was amazing. I decided that even though I didn't know anything about the military, it sounded like a good career for me.

I went to a recruitment center and spoke with a representative. He told me about the camaraderie that I would find in the Armed Forces and how great a career it would be. Finally, I felt like I found the thing that would make me happy. Where my strengths would be valued and where I could form true friendships. I'm excited to be training to become an artillery gunner.

I joined the Army because I want to help people and to serve my country. I want to be part of something meaningful. And I want to make my parents proud.

I chose artillery because I respect the power of weapons and because I was told I'm too small to be infantry. I love the thought of being able to protect my unit by being behind the guns, if I can't be on the front lines.

I joined the Army because, well, I feel like I've been training to fight my whole life.

I scratch things out and rewrite the answers about three times. When I finally finish writing, my stomach is growling, and I march to the meal hall. Halfway down the corridor, an officer monitoring a stopwatch stands beside a soldier on the floor holding plank. He yells at a group of us marching by: "Does everybody see what happens when you're caught walking instead of marching?" The guy in plank looks like he's in serious pain.

His unit marches around him in support, and I join them and ask, "How long has he been there?"

"Ten minutes so far."

"For not marching?"

"Yep. If you don't want to be that guy, you better march. No matter what."

Rule number three.

The long tables, noisy chatter, and clink of utensils in the meal hall make me feel like I'm back in high school, deciding whom to sit with.

"Hi, I'm Kelsi." I slide my tray into the last spot at a full table. "Hey," says the guy across from me.

"Your first night?" says another.

"You can tell?"

They all laugh. "You didn't get your meal card punched," adds a girl farther down. "If you don't, you get in trouble. They want to make sure you're eating three meals a day."

"Thanks." That's rule number four. I take a big bite of my pizza. It's a favorite around here, and I won't have an issue punching my card today.

"Where'd you go to school?" asks the guy next to me.

"St. Mary's Secondary and Campbellford District High School. You?"

"Guelph University."

"So why'd you join?" I ask him.

"Piss off my parents. I'm infantry. You?"

"Artillery."

A guy across from me smirks. "I'm Navy."

A young guy with a buzz cut calls out, "Go Army, beat Navy!"

Another guy stands up and stacks his food tray. "Have fun sleeping in the mud and throwing up over the side of a boat. Air Force tops all of you!"

"Army beats Navy."

"Dirty seamen!" Everyone starts to laugh.

The teasing and trash-talking put me at ease. It's been less than twenty-four hours, and already I'm connecting with people, just like the Armed Forces rep told me would happen. The quiet in my dorm made me uncomfortable, but now I feel I'm in the right place and that I made the right decision.

Later, when I enter my room, in the silence among strangers, apprehension returns. I wonder what tomorrow has in store for me. By the time I crawl into my cot, underneath stiff, starched sheets and an itchy wool blanket, I'm excited and terrified at the same time.

A pounding on the door wakes me. A collective groan sweeps across the entire room, but I can't even make a sound yet. I hear some yelling in the distance and hope the racket stops so I can doze off again.

Our main door is kicked open. "Get up!"

With one eye open, I look at the time. I'm a morning person, but 0400 comes real early when you're not ready for it. There's screaming and yelling from the hallway, then loud footsteps.

"Get out! Get out!"

I haven't been out of bed this early since I was training for my black belt, and suddenly I'm thankful for those eight years of early morning practices. I roll out of bed as the sergeant marches toward my end of the room.

"Move it! Down the stairs! Now!"

My whole troop exits like a stream of fish toward the door, where people are tripping over their feet, pushing into the hall, and rumbling down the stairs. On the main floor, there's a semblance of calm and a chorus of yawns as we stand obediently in a line.

Half of us aren't fully awake as the sergeant paces in front of us. "It's time for physical training. PT! Every morning from now on, you're to be ready at 0400. I'm not your mommy coming to wake you." He glares down the line, and I'm sure his eyes pause on me for a moment. "You are to be fed, dressed, downstairs, and waiting together in two perfect lines. If one of you is late, or you're down here with unpolished boots, everyone is treated to an extra round of push-ups or an extra mile outside in the cold." His voice hardens. "There will be consequences."

Rule number five: One person screws up, we all screw up, and we will all pay for it together. Maybe the *only* rule that really matters.

February 2008

There's something peaceful about running in the early morning when your feet crunch in the snow, your breath rises in the frosty air, and your nose hairs freeze in the cold. I'm the first of the girls to finish the 10K run, and I could easily do another 5K, but it's time to march to breakfast before getting cleaned up and ready for inspection.

I've been an athlete my entire life, and the physical challenges here are nothing new to me. Black belts don't come for free. Give me more running, more push-ups, more sit-ups, more chin-ups, the biggest sandbags. Give me a heavier kit. Push me harder. I know it isn't a competition, and we need to be training as a unit, but this stuff comes naturally to me. I was built for it.

We're now six weeks into training, and some people have dropped out. I've tried helping some of my troop, but they don't want it. So while we're here to be "stronger together than apart," I also make it my mission to be stronger than anyone else. I'm the smallest person here, but that is nothing new to me either. This is just another challenge, and thanks to Mom and Dad drilling it into my head that I can do anything if I work hard enough, I'm mentally prepared to deal with it.

At meal hall, I walk toward an empty seat at a table with a blonde girl from my room, but she quickly puts her jacket on the seat. I'll admit, I thought making friends would be easier than this. I continue to another table, where the rest of the girls from my room are, and I sit down with my tray.

"Hi."

They don't even look at me, so I dig into my eggs, bacon, and toast, barely chewing. Their behavior reminds me of a rugby tournament in Florida, and I'm transported back to my high school days:

"Check out mine!" One of the girls on my team passes around her new ID to the rest of my teammates while I stare out the window at the palm trees whizzing by. While I'm hoping the last Gravol I took—which is a medication I use to treat and prevent motion sickness as well as nausea, vomiting, and dizziness—will hold me until we get to the hotel, all they can think of is partying.

"Oh my God! Yours totally looks real."

"I can't believe we didn't get caught!" whispers one of them.

"I know! Last night was epic."

I'm away from my parents for the first time, and while I was sleeping last night to be rested for the upcoming games, they all snuck out of the hotel to get belly button piercings and fake IDs. I am so ready to graduate and get out of Campbellford. These girls accept me because I score for the team, but I will never be one of them.

It doesn't feel a lot different here. Maybe I should try harder, but I'm not sure what to do. I'll ask Mom about it when I see her and Dad in a couple of days. Everything seemed so new and promising at the beginning of basic, but it's been a long six weeks. I don't want to burden Mom, since I know it will be a long drive for my parents to get here, but I just can't wait to talk to people who genuinely like me. I need this visit. I look up at my troop with another attempt. "I'm starving after PT."

"Gonna show us up in eating, too?"

One of the girls sneers. "I'll just go bang out twenty-five chin-ups in a row."

"I've been doing them since I was a kid in martial arts. I can show you a trick that works for me," I offer, but instead of accepting my gesture, they turn their attention to a bunch of guys at the next table that are joking around. One of the guys is turning into a goddamned super soldier, which, frankly, pisses me off. His marching is smoother, his beret is shaped better, his boots are shinier, his rifle is perfect, his PT is on point, and he crushes the social game of BMQ (Basic Military Qualification) life.

I want to be him. Calm, cool, collected; but the women treat me like I'm a bitch.

The seat beside the blonde is still empty. Clearly, she was giving me a message. Despite my efforts, things aren't getting any better; in fact, the tenser that training gets, the more tired and stressed everyone is, the less I'm making friends.

The BS I thought I left in high school followed me to college and here, too, apparently. Anyway, I'm training for my career, not to win a popularity contest, so the hell with 'em. Part of me actually enjoyed the shit talking. It meant that they viewed me as strong. And it gave me fuel to wipe the floor with them.

After breakfast, I march to my room. I'm going to make good and sure my chore is done perfectly, because I don't feel like holding a push-up position for a half hour or getting us grounded this weekend. The floors are already clean enough to eat off of, but I scrub again anyway. When I enter the bathroom, I see a drip trailing from the bar of soap into the sink. What's going on? Nobody has started to clean in here yet? I step out of the room. "Hey, it's almost time for inspection, which of you is on bathroom today?"

"Oh, we're not doing it." One of them removes a clump of hair from her brush and watches it drop onto the floor.

"You have to," I remind her. "We will lose our Saturday if we don't pass inspection, and the week before was the first time we were allowed to leave since getting here."

"Exactly," they chime in. "We'll all get in trouble if it's not done, so you'll do it, Burns."

There's no point in fighting with them. I'm the teenager here, and it's the thirty- and forty-year-old women I'm living with who are acting like children. They're right. They don't care, and they know I'll do it. With a glare, I pick up her hair from the floor, turn, and rush back to the bathroom. All the while, they're laughing at me. Six more weeks of this. Six more weeks.

While I'm finishing the floors, scrubbing the toilet, and rinsing the sink, I focus on getting a bear hug from Dad, seeing Mom's smile, and telling them about my training. There are so many things I can't wait to share, like swim training and how much "fun" it is to tread water in full uniform—including boots—holding weights. Everyone better have their shit together for inspection so we get our weekend. I do a quick check around the pod and make sure everything's inspection-ready then hurry back to my bunk. I open my drawers; everything's in place. My socks have been painstakingly rolled and folded into one another like little wool envelopes. I check my bed for the proper forty-five-degree-angle folds in the sheets. My boots are shined. My rifle is clean. Everything else on my mental checklist seems to be good. I want to smack the others, but I'm good.

The sergeant's boots thump as he enters our pod, so I adjust my feet, quickly check that my hair is tucked under my beret, and stand at attention. A breath of relief comes from everyone as he leaves our room. We're cleared!

But in a few minutes, I hear him yelling from the next room. Our staff is always yelling, but yelling during inspection is bad. I hear a thud and more yelling—someone got their pod flipped.

I take a deep breath and count to ten to stop myself from screaming. We just lost our Saturday, and now I have to spend the day with my unit doing more drills instead of hanging out with my parents. I lean against the wall and close my eyes to fight back the tears. My roommates are laughing. "Ah, poor little Burns misses her mommy and daddy," one of them jeers. "But thanks for cleaning the bathroom. You can do it again tomorrow."

A lump rises in my throat. I've never missed my parents like this, and now I have to call them and say I can't see them this weekend.

They came all this way for nothing.

An hour later, we're standing outside in rows of four for bayonet rifle training. All I can hear is the disappointed sound of my parents' voices, and my anger grows. I get the point: One of us messes up, everyone suffers, but I'm still pissed off. Following orders precisely is a critical lesson when you're preparing for war. A pencil out of place on a desk is a preventable error. They told us how to do it, and we have to do what they say. One preventable mistake in combat equals death. One person makes a little blunder, everyone dies.

After a few hours, I'm chilled to the bone, even though I'm in my full winter uniform: thermal underwear, thermal undershirt, polar fleece pants, polar fleece shirt, combat toque, combat parka, parka bib pants, gloves, wool socks, and mukluk boots. The snow has started melting, but the ground is frozen and icy. I can barely feel my feet.

I bring my rifle to my chest for the millionth time today as we wait for the order.

"FIX BAYONET!"

A succession of clicks rings out as we unsheathe our bayonets, sun glinting off the metal blades, snapping them in place on our rifles. I no longer have to use my brain for this drill. My muscles know what to do, and this is what they want.

I step forward and lunge, rifle extended. Step back. Forward march, bring the rifle to my side. Again and again. I stand back up, screaming, "KILL!" and with everyone else, I jab my rifle into the dummy's chest. Neutralizing the enemy.

Who the enemy is or where we will be facing him someday, I don't know, but we're told this training may save our lives.

THE WATCHER

Hello, Kelsi.

You haven't met me yet, but you will.

And I already know everything about you.

I've been logging details about your life since you almost died in the womb.

No wonder you're always so worried about doing things wrong. You couldn't even be born right.

Fun fact. The bullying will never stop for you.

That's what happens when you're weak.

TWO

Training

February 2008

My feet sink into the deep snow on our march into Farnham Training Camp. I keep pace as we trudge together in two lines, fully kitted up for a week "outside the wire."

It's our first training session beyond the confines of the secure military base. As we grind our way against a strong wind, I adjust my rucksack and push through the discomfort of carrying my own body weight while slogging in the snow. Farnham is the camp near Garrison used for field exercises, and we're promised a week-long "adventure" that involves subzero camping, sleep deprivation, reconnaissance missions on foot, and a timed 13k ruck march. I keep my eyes peeled, watching for any sign of the "enemy" hiding in the trees, knowing we could be ambushed at any time.

"Why do you seem so paranoid, Burns?" one of the guys behind me shouts.

"Staff is watching us like hawks and evaluating us," I call out. "Right now. Even when cleaning our kit."

"Not when we're sleeping and eating." He laughs. "I'm looking forward to sentry duty. You?"

"QRF." I can't wait for quick reaction force. "The rest of this week is going to suck, but we're almost done."

We reach a clearing in the woods with a cluster of little wooden sheds and break up into groups of eight.

"I want to be one of the snipers," says the guy with a lisp.

"So, my brother did this," adds the tattooed guy with a knowing grin. "Lots of walking the fence of the compound, watching the gate, sitting up in the tower and looking out for any signs of suspicious activity."

"Can't imagine having more fun," chimes another.

"They just want you to obey every order." The tattooed guy snaps his heels together. "March, clean, shoot, eat, sleep." He points at us. "Obey, don't question, and you stay alive."

"Where's your brother deployed to now?"

"Afghanistan."

"It's brutal there, I heard." The guy with the lisp opens the door to the shelter.

"My brother says no amount of training prepared him for it. That you can't imagine unless you've been there."

"But it's helping the people there, right?" asks another.

"Yeah, but it's no peace mission. My brother says the Taliban is everywhere. It's full-on war."

I follow the group into the shelter, wondering what actual war will be like. The sweet scent of chipboard greets us. I can see my breath and a thin layer of ice on the window. The moment I sit down on the cot, my heavy rucksack slides off my back. This pack contains everything I'll need, from underwear, air mattress, and sleeping bag to a gas mask, helmet, and a flashlight. When my face has thawed enough for me to speak, I ask, "Did your brother say if we get one good night's sleep?"

He shakes his head, and before he can answer fully, above the muffled sound of the roaring wind, we hear, "Mealtime."

"Tonight's the last hot meal," one of the guys says, grinning ear to ear.

"Yeah." Another nods. "Tomorrow it's good old bomb-proof ration packs."

"I don't mind rations," adds the tattooed guy. "Some of them are actually pretty good."

"Any idea who the enemy is in the simulations?" asks another.

"My brother said you never know. And it doesn't matter. Our lives could be snuffed out at any point, and it could be by a kid, a woman, a man. We kill them and protect each other; that's all that matters in war."

After supper, as I burrow into my sleeping bag, I think about his brother's comment. If this was real, and I was now deployed with these seven guys, our lives would depend on each other. I'm in my cot, fully dressed except for my boots, ready to show them they can count on me.

I bolt awake about an hour after lights-out to banging, yelling, and the whistle pop of gunfire. Game time.

We scramble out of our cots and into our boots.

"What'd I tell you!" the guy with the lisp shouts through his hood. We grab our weapons and race outside to the gates of our makeshift base, breaking up into our troops of four. Hunched against the strong wind while getting into position, I'm both exhilarated and exhausted but glad that I went to bed in my combat parka. Even though my teeth chatter and my feet ache, my old friend adrenaline is alive and slowly warming me up.

ADRENALINE

There's a little flaw in your training here.

They keep warning you about the enemy, but when you're faced with the Taliban, they won't be holding up signs or wearing badges to identify themselves.

Every single person with brown skin is someone who might kill you.

You'll find that out soon enough when you're done playing pretend war.

February 2008

The next morning, I choke down "sausage and hash browns" from a brown envelope before we hit the range for our shooting lesson. Rations taste amazing when you're exhausted and hungry.

Pulling my toque down tighter on my head, I cover my ears against the cold and the sound of the rifles firing downrange. I shuffle my feet to send some warmth into my body, until, finally, it's my turn to shoot. Moving quickly, we trade our hats for helmets and put on our eye protection.

My boots crunch in the snow as I take my place at the platform. As I lift the gun, my hands tremble. I signed up to be an artillery gunner, and I've never fired a weapon before. Narrowing my eyes on the target I'm aiming for, I follow the officer's instructions, racking the weapon, pulling the butt against my right shoulder, right hand on the trigger, left hand on the barrel. Nervous energy runs through me as I look into the sight of the rifle and line up for my shot.

Staff is on the lookout to see which of us might make a good sniper; I'm just hoping to hit the target. I pull the trigger and the bullet charges down the range, a brass casing flies out behind me, and I hit my target. The power in that shot sends a jolt of excitement through me as the scent of fresh gunpowder lingers in my nose.

I continue to shoot, and each time it's less intimidating. One of the other girls here, Sara-Lynn, gets the marksmanship awards. She's bad-ass and I'm proud of her. After she's named the winner, I approach her. "Hey, congratulations. You did awesome."

"Thanks. You did great, too."

"I'll take pointers from you anytime." I pull my hat tighter.

"You're on. I heard you're a black belt, so show me a thing or two." "Anytime, but right now I'm starving. Want to eat lunch together?"

Sara-Lynn nods as we walk to a quieter area. We rip into our rations, both of us too hungry to talk or even care about what we're eating.

"Which trade are you?" I gulp down my last bite.

"Navy," she manages between mouthfuls. "I want to be a medic."

"Cool. I'm Army. Artillery gunner."

"Battle drills and formations are next." She shuffles her feet to warm up. "You'll ace that one!"

By the end of the day, I'm mentally and physically exhausted from the amount of activity my body has been through, the new information I'm taking in, and the lack of sleep. My feet are soaking wet, and my heels are starting to blister from rubbing against my boots. I maneuver into my sleeping bag and close my eyes, looking forward to a bit of rest for my brain and my body.

I'm almost asleep when the door flies open with the sergeant screaming, "Get out of bed now!"

We pull our boots on as we jump out of bed. "Do you all think this is a joke?" He's pacing around the room, knocking over chairs.

"Do you understand what happens if someone falls asleep when they aren't supposed to? People fucking die! Someone in your unit fell asleep during their two-hour sentry duty shift, and now you all pay. Get your rifles and start running."

We dash into the darkness, slip-sliding in the ice-cold rain. He's not wrong. If you sleep when you're responsible for watching and protecting your entire unit, the enemy will be watching, and they'll wipe you all out. People will die. *Your* people. The people you train with, work with, become family with.

"I hate Sarge," says the guy with the lisp.

"Exactly what they want," yells the tattooed guy as he runs past us. "Break you down emotionally and physically."

I run after him, away from all the bitching and moaning. When you make a mistake like that, you can't take it back.

We run and run and run until people start dropping like flies and the staff can see we've been pushed hard enough. We're sent back to bed.

But we're woken up twenty minutes later by another kick at the door. "QRF ON ME!"

I jump up, scramble to my feet, grab my weapon, and race out the door. Finally! It's QRF time. This is where things get fun as we learn what it will be like in an actual war zone.

Gunfire rings out in the pitch black, and I run with my unit toward the sound.

There's a flash in the dark—the muzzle of an enemy's rifle—and we all duck into a ditch for cover.

Rain pours down around my helmet, and I shiver as I unclip my night-vision goggles and put them on. Everything looks green, but at least I'm not completely blind out here in the dark. My blood pumps hard, pushing adrenaline through my veins. We have no idea what we're running into, and I love it. This is what we will face in war, and this is the training that will count. These are the drills we hope are good enough to keep us alive.

In an instant, we're overrun by the enemy. They're running around soaking wet, dressed in jeans and flannel shirts with masks on—riot gear to mimic what we may face in guerrilla warfare. My unit rushes forward, shouting and screaming. No sooner do I grab one than he hits me in the abdomen. I see the second blow coming. No way am I going to let the enemy win! I strike first, grip his hands behind his back, and push him forcefully to his knees.

"Gas, gas, GAS!"

Shit!

I tie the guy's hands together and unclip the bag containing my protective gear from my belt. Quickly, I pull on my gas mask and climb into my suit before dragging my prisoner into the barn, where we are corralling them for their "protection."

I run into the darkness, pummel another enemy, and haul him over to the barn.

"Burns, are you using too much force?" the guy with the lisp calls out.

"He's the enemy!" I bark back.

"We're under attack," shouts the tattooed guy as he shoves his prisoner ahead. "We don't have time to debate right and wrong.

You're here to protect your troop and gun down the enemy." He pushes his prisoner into the barn. "That's what soldiers do."

He's right. The enemy isn't giving up, and if this was war and it was down to hand-to-hand combat, the outcome of losing would be death.

I have never lost well.

February 2008

I swear to God, I will never take dry feet for granted again.

On kilometer eight million of our thirteen-kilometer ruck march, my heavy pack feels like five hundred, and we're not allowed to run. However, we can do the airborne shuffle, dragging your feet in basically a light jog, and I am an expert at that. Me and my little legs. I land strangely on my left foot, and a little reminder of pain shoots through the bones.

Suddenly my mind takes me back to Tae Kwon Do class: I'm crumpled on the mat, a man standing over me. My foot burns. I felt it crack. I don't want to look at it.

The man pokes and prods me. Is he a doctor? Maybe. Whoever he is, whatever he's doing, it hurts. He's saying words, but I'm not listening. All I can think about is my black belt. "Ouch!" He mumbles an apology and gets up to talk to Coach.

I'm only halfway through day one of the two-day testing. I know my patterns and I can pass this part. I'm not worried about tomorrow, either, the sparring and self-defense, but I need my feet. I scan the gym and watch my friends going through their patterns. Each time I hear the snapping of their *doboks*, I hate them all. My goal is to get my black belt before I turn twelve, and I want it today. I can't let someone else in my club get theirs before me.

Mom plops a bag of ice on my feet. "Everything will be okay." Coach ambles toward us. I hope he has good news. Everything he says to me I take as gospel. When he speaks, it's like God is talking directly to me. I'll do what he says. I always do.

"So, Kelsi, you broke one foot and injured the other."

No!

"What now?" Mom asks.

"You have two choices. Nationals are around the corner, and you're fighting for the championship there. You don't need a black belt for that. You can either stop now and wait until you heal to test again, or freeze-spray and tape your feet and go for it."

My feet are swelling up and one's turning blue. I turn to Mom. "What should we do?"

She shrugs. "You have to decide, kiddo. I'm not going to be the reason you don't get your belt or why you can't fight at nationals."

The ice has numbed my foot, but the second I try to wiggle my toes, pain shoots straight to my ankle. I have the rest of today to get through, and tomorrow's going to be even harder. Can I do this? I look at my mom and think of everything she's given up to get me to this point in my training. I turn to my coach. "Tape 'em up."

With my first kick, I wonder if I made the right decision, but I push through. My uniform snaps with every kick as I work through my patterns. I feel my feet swelling and bruising under the tape, but I push through it. Every few minutes, pain sends goosebumps down my arms and legs.

You're almost done... Almost done...

I'm sore, but I get through it.

Day two. I start with self-defense and fight someone double my size.

At this point, my busted feet don't even affect me—adrenaline is a beautiful thing. But now it's time for sparring. If I want to make it to the end, I'm going to have to kick people over and over for the rest of the day, using a lot of force. With cracked and broken feet.

I get through my one-on-one sparring and then I hear an announcement, "Now we will move to two-on-one."

I'm trying to focus on my form and fight off two people while instinctively protecting my feet. Coach and Mom cheer me on, but I can't feel my toes, and a searing pain keeps reminding me that I have a broken bone. I shouldn't have done this. I'm going to screw my chances at nationals. My muscles ache. My eyes fill with tears. I can't do this anymore.

Mom and Coach cheer, "You're almost done. You almost have it. You've got this, Kelsi!"

I take a deep breath, and I'm back. I'm kicking, I'm blocking, I'm punching, and that's it. The whistle blows. It's over.

I feel like I'm moving in slow motion as I make my way to the bench. Mom has me in a hug. Coach is patting my back. Teammates are cheering for me.

I made it through something I didn't think possible. I'm a second degree black belt in Tae Kwon Do.

If could do that, this hell march that I'm currently slogging my way through should be nothing. But by kilometer nine, I'm about to give up from exhaustion when an angel named Lieutenant (LT) Labonté runs up beside me. "Burns, keep pushing."

"I'm trying!"

She matches my stride. She isn't a lot bigger than me or a lot older, and she has a warm, friendly face. In another world, we would be friends.

"I know you can do it. Keep going."

"I'm so tired. It's so cold."

"Listen, I'll give you some chocolate if you finish this kilometer."

"Okay," I say, panting. I push my legs to their limits and get it done in time.

As promised, LT Labonté reaches into her pocket and pulls out a mini chocolate bar, handing it to me. There's a twinkle in her eye when she quietly says in her thick French accent, "Look how many of the guys you beat."

This feeling is sweeter than all the chocolate in the world, but it doesn't last long, because immediately after the march, it's time for the fireman's carry. Being the smallest person here, I'm at a big disadvantage, but I'm running on adrenaline. I'm paired with a girl only a couple inches taller than me. I can do this. From a squat position, I pick her up with my right arm and drape her awkwardly over my

27

shoulder. I right-foot-left-foot march myself through the burning in my calves and thighs, and I'm finished before my time's up.

Finally, there's the trench dig. My feet are numb, but this day has been 100 percent absolute crap, and it's all about mind over matter. It's where my martial arts training kicks in.

"Remind me why I signed up for this?" whimpers the guy with the lisp.

I'm too tired even to think about that, and I just keep turning over my shovel in the semi-frozen ground. They're making us do this for a reason, so I keep digging.

"Just a few more weeks till graduation," grunts the tattooed guy. "They're just reprogramming us through the tiredness in training. It's all just a game."

A GAME

It's nice to see military training hasn't changed.

Just a big, elaborate game.

They instruct you to follow orders without questioning.

They break you down to build you up, all the while training you to fight the enemy you can see.

Neglecting to warn you about the one you can't.

That's why I have an advantage, and I will always win.

THREE

Weapons Handling

I'm doodling in the margins of my notebook when the teacher sets the box of Timbits mini doughnuts—our class reward—on my desk. "Which one would you like, Kelsi?"

The smell of chocolate tempts me momentarily. I can't remember the last time I had something as bad as a doughnut. "Kelsi won't have one of those," one of my classmates says. "She doesn't eat junk food. I'll have hers."

Without looking up, I keep drawing patterns within the lines of the paper. If I could eat that kind of thing, I'd definitely take a chocolate one, and I would eat it in five bites. Maybe after the tournament. "I can't have one."

"Why not?"

"I have to lose weight."

"Don't be silly," the teacher whispers. "You're tiny as it is."

I shake my head. "Nationals are next week, and I have to make weight."

She removes the box from my desk and moves on to the next kid. I consider turning around and checking to see if there was a chocolate one left, but I don't. I stay strong.

29

When I get home from school, I drop my backpack on the floor and head straight for the kitchen, grabbing an apple from the bowl on the counter and crunching into it.

"Kelsi?" I can tell by the tone in Mom's voice that she isn't happy about something.

"Yeah?"

"I got a call from the principal today."

"Why? I didn't do anything."

"Did your teacher hand out doughnuts today?"

"Yeah." I take another bite of my apple, juice dripping down my chin.

"Did you say you couldn't have one because you have to lose weight?"

"Yeah."

"You know a Timbit isn't going to make a difference."

"We're flying to Vancouver in a week, and I have to make weight. I'm not jeopardizing my training for a piece of gross deep-fried batter."

Mom takes a deep breath. "Well, now your teacher is afraid that you're starving yourself."

"I'm not!"

"I know that. But I've gone ahead and called the doctor to get you checked out just to make sure you're at a healthy weight."

"All I did was refuse a doughnut."

"But it's not normal for a seventy-pound twelve-year-old girl to refuse a doughnut because she's trying to lose weight. I'm starting to worry about why there aren't any signs of puberty yet, too."

"God, Mom. Fine. I'll go to the doctor and prove I'm not malnourished."

April 2008

Given my size, during my four weeks of weapon training, the Carl Gustav Rocket Launcher is the biggest challenge, and I'd eat a box of Timbits if it would help me. Carl G can be fired from most positions:

sitting, kneeling, standing, lying on the ground, and it takes two people to shoot it. Or three Kelsi-sized people. The launcher weighs a good thirty pounds, and one person carries and fires it while the other hauls and loads the ammo. At four feet long, it can fire somewhere between four hundred and two thousand meters, depending on the circumstances.

Carl G is no joke.

To keep this crazy machine steady, I hold it on my right shoulder with my right hand on the trigger and my left holding a handle beneath the barrel. Another woman stands to my right, helping me balance the weapon.

We wait for the command: "Load!"

My partner puts the rocket in the chamber while I keep the weapon aimed at the target. "Load!" she shouts.

A sergeant comes over and wraps his arms around us to keep us stable while we shoot.

Then comes the next command: "Ready!"

We brace ourselves for the kickback that's sure to come. I've never fired a rocket before, and I'm excited! "Ready!" we shout.

"Range 250. Reference target number one!"

We repeat the order, and I'm full of adrenaline. Finally comes the best command: "FIRE!"

"Fire!"

I squeeze the trigger, and my partner and I tremble in the wake of the rocket as it zooms downrange, landing on our target. I feel my entire brain shake, as if I just got kicked in the head, the snot comes running out my nose. That fucking rocked my brain.

After spending so much time underneath the Carl G, my hands vibrate, my hearing is muffled, and my legs are like rubber. The machine guns are next, and I feel like Rambo. There's enough power in my index finger when I'm holding one of these to take out an entire enemy unit. Inexperienced hands should never touch machine guns. Hell, they should never be used outside of a military situation. I can't believe we only get four weeks of training on these things. I want to understand how to use them properly, and I don't want to get cocky with them. The margin for error here is zero. They are capable of mass destruction, and I respect that power.

EXPLOSIVES

Remember this thought, Kelsi.

You'll laugh at it one day.

Or not.

March 2008

My arms burn, and the black flies assault my face as my pickax bounces off the rocks. It's our fourth and final week of DP1 (Developmental Period 1) and we're on another training exercise, similar to Farnham. Fan-fucking-tastic.

Day after day we've gone through practice maneuvers till the muscle memory is strong, and I feel like I can operate one of these guns in my sleep. I'm stronger than I've ever been after handling the heavy ammo rounds, but this exercise is wearing me down.

"Feels like I'm digging my own grave."

My partner grunts and jabs at the ground. We are going to be attacked at some point by the "enemy" here, just as we were in Farnham; but this time, we will be far more sleep-deprived. We aren't permitted to sleep tonight, but this terrain will keep us from it anyway. Rocks, more rocks, hard-packed clay, and rocks.

I push my helmet up over my eyes, but it slides back down on a glistening layer of sweat. Pain sears into my palms as a blister bursts. It's the second one, even though I'm wearing gloves. I swat at gnats and black flies as they swarm around my nostrils and in my ears, and then I pound my pickax into the ground. Two pieces fly into the air.

"Burns!" Sergeant yells.

"Goddammit! I—" The flies swarm into my mouth, and I snatch my new pickax from his hand. More black flies crawl around my neck, and I smack at them as I march back to my spot.

By the time we can stand in our hole, it's as dark as the sky. I wouldn't call it a trench yet, but I require less hole to hide in than my six-foot-tall fire mission buddy, so it works for me.

I recede as far as possible underneath the hood of my jacket, escaping the black flies and running my hands over the large welts they've chewed into my neck.

"BURNS!" Sergeant's voice sears in my eardrums. My eyes blink open, and I claw at the earth to get my bearings.

"You just KILLED your fire team partner!" he screams. The veins are popping on his neck.

The words make my stomach turn, and I can't even look over at my buddy. I fell asleep when I was supposed to be watching. If we were in war, I would be responsible for the death of my comrades. I will never let my partner down again.

LOSER

You're messing up, Kelsi.

Just like I want.

Good girl.

You're not sure what day it is anymore.

You'll never make it in Afghanistan!

You've only been awake for seventy-two hours, and your mind is already playing tricks on you.

I love seeing your eyes wobble so you start to see things that aren't there.

That's it, Kelsi, close your eyes against the black flies.

Close them just long enough to fall asleep, you loser.

The sound of gunfire in the early morning scares the crap out of everyone. I jump up to see what's going on, and the sergeant is firing an entire twenty-eight-round clip in the trench, screaming at one of the guys, "Everyone is dead because of YOU! Because you couldn't do one thing, STAY AWAKE TO PROTECT YOUR TROOP!" He stomps toward the soldier who was sleeping and hands back the rifle. "DO YOU UNDERSTAND?"

He glares at the rest of us. "YOU ARE ALL FUCKING DEAD!" he yells and stomps toward all of us. "When you're on watch, you open your eyes and stay awake."

I'm now more awake than I have ever been in my entire life, and I channel all of that anxious energy into our 13k ruck march. I'm kitted up and ready to do this testing all over again in the field. I trudge along the trail, feeling the fifty pounds on my back and my lack of sleep during the last five days. Adrenaline carries me on the first five kilometers, and I feel good. My body understands what I need it to do because we've done this before. Is it going to suck? Hell yes. But I'll finish with a bit of mind over matter and some sheer stubbornness.

This mentality carries me through twelve kilometers, and then my feet are on fire. The pain swallows me, radiating up through my ankles to my knees. I feel like I'm losing my mind and stop midstride.

Come on, I chastise myself. *You can do this.*

Slowly I take another step. If I stop now, I'll have to start from the beginning, and that's not an option. I plod along the trail, counting out each step. Just when I start to slow down again, LT Labonté comes up behind me. "Come on, Burns!" she shouts. "You've got this."

She hands me some Swedish Berries, which she knows I love. I pop the sweet, chewy candies into my mouth and pick up my pace with the sugar kick.

"Finish and you'll get more."

"Okay, LT." I have it in me, and she believes in me. I don't want to let her down.

I continue marching on burning feet for candy, and somehow, I make it to the end.

My feet are screaming at me, but there's still a fireman's carry and trench dig ahead. I just have to put my head down, eat the pain, and do it. I've done it before.

By the time I finish, I have no strength left, but this part of the course is over. I have survived a week of sleep deprivation and grueling physical tasks, and now hot showers and rest await us.

"Start cleaning your weapons," says the sergeant as we get into the barracks.

"Then we're sleeping?"

"Not you! I am. Going home now, and then will be back tomorrow to make sure you're staying awake."

"And when do we sleep?"

"You don't. We're taking turns to go home and rest so someone is always awake to watch you."

I don't know if I can handle this. We are all too tired, but we have no choice. Other than a bit of food and water on the table for us, we're on our own and are in for more sleep deprivation. I can feel my will wavering.

The tattooed guy is so tired he passes out. Sergeant puts a helmet on him and then yells in his ear, "So you don't hurt yourself when you fall down!"

We all crack up laughing at this, because everything is hilarious after a week of no sleep.

After ten days of this, I've lost all sense of time, and that's when we are finally sent back to the barracks to rest. When I get to my pod, I untie my boots and grimace in pain as I pull them off my feet. I remove my socks, and the searing agony of peeling flesh brings me to tears.

"Medic!" I cry weakly.

"Your feet are wrecked, Burns," the medic says, examining me.

"No shit. It feels like a hangnail peeling down the center of my foot to my ankle."

"I need to bandage them up."

"How am I going to finish my training with my feet bandaged?"

"I don't think you can."

The hell with that. *Think, Kelsi. You need to find a way around this impossible problem.*

I squeeze my eyes shut and consider different solutions. I let my mind go back a couple of years; I've proven to the rugby coach that I'm good enough to make the cut and am desperate to be part of a team. "But, Burns," he says, "your academic average needs to go way up if you want to play."

"I can't get my marks any higher. I actually try my hardest as it is. I study and study, but math is like a foreign language."

"Try harder."

"I'll never get my average higher unless I can play sports all day and get graded on that." And then it hits me. "Coach, do physical fitness credits count?"

"Yep."

I remember that I aced a couple of phys-ed courses to bring my overall mark up high enough to make the team. There is always a workaround.

I call my sergeant over and point to my feet as they're getting bandaged up. "My boots won't fit. Can I complete the last part of my training in flip-flops?"

He turns to the medic. "How long?"

He shrugs. "Not sure, but she can get into running shoes soon and then work her way back into boots."

Sergeant nods. "Heal fast, Burns."

It means a lot that my staff knows how hard I've worked up to this point. I'm so thankful they aren't forcing me to start over.

Luckily, this week's exercises are doable in flip-flops, even though I look ridiculous, and within four days, I'm able to wear running shoes. On the final day of artillery training, I'm back in boots. For this exercise, I take off my cornflake cap badge that identifies me as a private and wait my turn to fire live ammunition downrange for the first time. Each person in our troop is in sync. We've been going through these motions and positions as if we've learned to dance around the gun. We are all soldiers and know the basics of our rifles, fighting, and military life to serve as infantry. And now this.

It's my turn to load my first live round.

I approach the howitzer and move over to the lanyard, waiting for the call. I'm locked and loaded, and when I hear the word, "Fire!" I wrap the lanyard in my hand, squeeze the absolute crap out of it, and pull it against my hips with a twist until I hear the loud boom. The projectile flies down the range toward a target ten kilometers away and hits it perfectly.

And with that, I earn my new artillery cap badge, am done with my training, and am now officially a gunner in the Canadian Armed Forces. More than that, though, I'm a gunner with the artillery. The cool thing is that I know how to run one of these huge guns and can protect a whole troop from forty kilometers away. I can't wait to tell Mom and Dad.

Later in the day, I find out I've been posted to Petawawa, Ontario. I'm happy that it will bring me closer to my parents, but I'm disappointed. I'm joining a unit that isn't deploying, and I want to go overseas, use my new skills, and fight.

So when the opportunity comes up to trade postings with someone who isn't healthy enough to deploy, I jump on it. I knock on LT Labonté's office door.

She looks up from her desk. "Hello, Burns. What is it?"

I take a step inside and blurt, "I hear there's a guy that's not able to go to Valcartier in Quebec. I would like to volunteer to trade postings with him."

"Sit down." She looks me straight in the eye. "You do realize that Valcartier is deploying to Afghanistan?"

I nod, and she waits a moment, letting me think it over. I wonder what Afghanistan will be like after all that we were told of fighting in a war, and all of our drills. Does she not think I'm ready? I think back to the times she offered me encouragement, the chocolates, the

Swedish Berries, and hope she doesn't think I'm not strong enough. My eyes move over the medals on her uniform, then to photos on the wall. I do not dream about killing people, but I am prepared to protect my guys.

"You're sure?" Her mischievous brown eyes are now thoughtful and warm.

"Yes, ma'am." I sit up straight in my chair and study her, trying to imagine what she's thinking. Whenever I needed a push, she was always there for me. She has to know that I want this more than anything.

"You're aware of the conflicts there?"

I nod, although I'm not really sure, but I know the military will brief me, as they've done in our training exercises. "I'm ready to use my training as soon as possible and do my country proud."

She leans forward and ponders for a moment. I curl my fingers around the thin fabric of my uniform and feel my insides squirm in a way they haven't done since that first day the sergeant yelled at me. After all the stressful months of mental and physical training, the exhausting sleep deprivation, I want to finally prove what I'm capable of.

"I'll start the paperwork, but I don't see there being a problem."

"Thank you, LT. I won't let you down."

Back in my bunk, I keep packing and preparing for graduation, but now I'm vibrating. I've spent months training, the military believes in my ability, and I'm actually joining a regiment that's deploying. I can't wait.

GOOD TRADE

Well done, Kelsi.

You're going to Afghanistan!

That works out well for both of us.

You get your chance to try and prove something, and I get the chance to take you down at the knees.

Win-win.

You think *you're* excited?

I can't wait.

FOUR

Posted

September 2008

Trust is all I can think about as I walk across the stage to formally enter my new life as an artillery gunner. I've trained with these people, and some of them will be on my unit when I deploy. Who will have my back, when the time comes?

I hear my parents cheering for me and try to spot them in a crowd filled with dignitaries and family members dressed in their Sunday best. When I see my Mom, Dad, and Dillon, I flash a smile. They have been there for me my whole life, supporting me in everything I have ever done, including making the trip all the way up here to watch me graduate. I am so happy they are here, but I am happier that basic training is over. Thank God.

After the ceremony, as I'm snapping photos with my family, I hear "Burns!" A staff member waves me and a couple other guys aside. "The five of you who will be going to Valcartier need to speak fluent French."

"Excuse me?"

"Few people there speak English, so you're going to need to learn fast."

Awesome.

I'm deploying with a 99 percent male unit, and I won't understand what they're saying. This is terrifying. But all I can do is learn the language.

FRENCH

I saw you in school.

I was there when you couldn't get through grade nine math on the second try.

You don't believe in your ability to learn another language at all, let alone in such a short time.

Let that feeling of self-doubt last a little bit longer.

It smells good on you.

September 16, 2008

"*Je voudrais du jus d'orange, des œufs et des saucisses s'il vous plaît*," I proudly tell the server.

"Your French has gotten so good!" my friend Bine cheers.

"*Merci*, Bine. All it took was you two helping to translate for me every single day for the past three months."

"*Bon anniversaire*, Kelsi." My other friend Jen raises her mug to mine.

I chuckle. "Yeah, it's my nineteenth birthday, and I sound like a five-year-old proudly ordering my breakfast *en français*!"

We all laugh and sip on coffee as we wait for our breakfast.

I am so happy right now with Bine and Jen, my two friends at Valcartier.

"It's nice to be away from those Valcartier assholes for a while," I declare. "That's a birthday gift in itself."

"Some of them are okay," Bine says.

"Yes, true. They aren't all bad," I admit.

"In fairness, you're not doing much to try to make friends with them," says Jen.

"You mean because I don't want to go out drinking with everyone?"

"Yeah, you know, that would help."

"Not happening. I'm not here to party. I'm here to train and go to war. Anyway, thank you for helping me. If I had to rely on the guys, I would never be able to speak French."

"Hey! You improved our English, too," Jen says.

"Well, I haven't had much luck with other women in basic, so thanks for not being dicks to me."

"They were just jealous. You nailed every challenge." Bine looks me straight in the eye. "You've got the kind of endurance soldiers dream of, and it comes natural to you."

"Cheers to that!" I raise my mug, and we all toast with our coffees.

"After the final round of training, the next time we see each other will be in Afghanistan." Jen takes a long sip.

"Yeah, it's crazy. I go home for a short visit, then meet with friends in Montreal, and then training in Alberta and Texas."

"Did you ever think it would happen so fast?" Bine looks out the window, then back at us. "I mean, all that training, and now we're going to be staring an enemy right in the eye."

"As long as it helps people." I sigh. "That's why I signed up. To be part of something meaningful."

I feel like I am exactly where I want to be in my life, and I don't have a care in the world, even though I'm literally getting ready to go to war.

* * *

After a quick visit home, I'm with friends at the Monster Energy after-party in Montreal, which they hold there each year, as sponsors of the Supercross series, pushing through the crowd of drunken people, one hand holding on to my high school friend, Elle, the other holding a beer. "It's time to go."

"Already?" she complains.

"Yeah. The Supercross race was epic, but things are getting out of hand."

"You're not that drunk."

"Drunk enough to know that if we stick around any longer, bad decisions are going to be made."

We're in no shape to drive, so we round up the rest of our group, hail a cab, and pile into a friend's hotel room. I'm ready to collapse into bed, but there is a problem: two beds and eight people. One bed has space left because the poor guy in it crashed his bike today, broke his wrist, and is trying to sleep.

Elle points at him. "If you squeeze in between me and that guy, we can sleep in that bed."

She doesn't want to sleep next to him because she has a boyfriend. "It's better than the floor, sure."

So we hop into bed, and this random guy turns toward me. "Hey, I'm Brady."

Damn. Tingles run down my spine. Can a spark actually feel like electricity? "Hey, I'm Kelsi."

"How was the party?"

His whole face lights up when he smiles.

"It was pretty crazy. Definitely lived up to the hype."

He's about my age, and from this angle, he seems to be a few inches taller than me.

"How's your wrist?"

"It doesn't feel awesome, but broken bones come with the job."

"Can you two be quiet? We're trying to sleep," someone from the other side of the room yells.

"How long have you been racing?" I whisper.

We smirk like children caught misbehaving. Brady motions toward my phone, opens up my BlackBerry Messenger app, and enters his info, then hands the phone back to me. I smile at him and send him a text:

How long have you been racing?

As he texts me back, I can't help but stare at him. He is gorgeous. I think I was supposed to meet him. My phone buzzes with his reply:

Since I was a kid.
  Cool. I get how sports can be tough on the body. I was an athlete as a kid, too.
  Oh yeah?
  Taekwondo, soccer, rugby...
  Where are you from? With your accent I assume not Quebec?
  Ha, no. A small town, Campbellford, Ontario. You?
  Vancouver.

Ah, crap. I want to get to know him much, *much* better, but geographically, even when and if I do make it back from Afghanistan, the distance will never work.

We continue texting for a couple of hours, and I fall asleep feeling like I may have just met the man I'm going to marry.

When I wake up at 0700, he's already gone. My heart sinks a bit, but when I pick up my phone, I see that he texted me: *By the way, you're cute when you're sleeping.*

Wainwright, Alberta, Fall 2008

Slowly, I open my eyes after sleeping well for the first time all week. When I try to sit up, my body doesn't move. My arms are stuck to my sides, and my legs won't budge. "I can't move! What's going on?" Rocking back and forth, I hear laughter and look down. I've been duct taped to my cot, and a quick scan of my surroundings tells me someone carried me out to the guns.

"Funny, guys. You're hilarious. Now help me out of here."

A prank in the military means acceptance, so I'm weirdly flattered. Annoyed, but it could be worse. At least I got some sleep. What we learn here at the giant training base in rural Alberta will go a long way toward keeping us alive when we deploy. It's heavy stuff, so laughter is appreciated from time to time.

When the opportunity arises, I text Brady—we've been exchanging messages back and forth since the night we met—to tell him the story. He sends me a *lol* and says *be careful*. This playful text relationship we have going is a very welcome distraction.

FLIRT

> A long-distance relationship is a great idea for you, Kelsi.
>
> A chance to put yourself out there, make yourself vulnerable, and then have your heart broken.
>
> I like it.

Me and another guy are with the guns, behind the trucks, on convoy to a new location for our course. We see a huge cloud of smoke billowing out of one of the trucks ahead of us. A voice comes over the radio, "*QRF pour troupe A!*"

That's me.

Grabbing my C7, I fasten my helmet and jump out of the truck to wait for my sergeant. He runs over. "Look out for anyone in the fields alongside us. The Taliban can be watching from there. If there's an IED—improvised explosive device—ahead, and it blows someone up, they'll film it and use it for propaganda."

"Disgusting."

"They're monsters, Burns."

"Makes me want to fight them and protect my guys even more."

Scanning the wide-open fields through my scope, I look for anyone with a radio, a cell phone, or some other sort of trigger device. Nothing. Walking to the rest of my team, I stop when a rope tied to a bush catches my gaze. Moving casually, careful not to arouse suspicion, I approach the rope. Someone could be watching me— someone with a trigger device.

"*Ne bouge pas!*" I whisper-yell to the guys ahead of me. *Don't move.*

They hear me and freeze.

When I finally reach them, a nod of my head toward the suspicious rope gets their attention.

Sergeant sees it now, too.

We get down good and low, crouching down through the frozen field, following the rope. It leads us out several meters, and there, at end of the rope, is a radio and an actor playing the enemy.

"Well done, Burns," says the sergeant. "You just spotted a secondary device."

"What does that mean?"

"The enemy set off the first device to mimic an explosion. Then, like fucking predators, they wait in the field like this, until a group rushes in to help the victims; then they use a secondary device to take out everyone."

"That's awful."

"These people are heartless, and they don't care about human life. Tactics like this are commonly used by the Taliban. If this were a real war situation, you would have saved your unit and helped to neutralize the enemy."

My training is making me sharp, and I'm getting more excited about deployment as the days go on. I am, however, aware that people on the other side of the world are training right now to take *me* out. This is just reality, and one that I'm coming to terms with. I have to trust my unit. I have to trust my country. But for some reason, when I fall asleep in my bunk during these training days, I keep waking up to the same memory. It's not one a want to relive, but it's one that keeps coming back.

* * *

The memory always starts the same way. My arms extend over my head in a big stretch, and I roll over and check the time on my alarm clock: 7:15 a.m.? *Oh, no! I slept in.*

I push the covers off myself and jump out of bed, bursting out my bedroom door. "Mom! Why did you let me sleep so late?"

46

I race to the kitchen and find Mom and Dad sitting at the table, drinking coffee. "Kelsi—" Mom starts to get up when she sees me. "I made pancakes."

"What's going on? Why did you let me sleep? I can't make it to the Olympics if I miss Tae Kwon Do practice!"

"No Tae Kwon Do today." Dad takes a sip of coffee.

"Why not? You wouldn't let me go last night, either!"

"Don't worry about why. You're not going, and that's that." Dad gets up from the table to pour more coffee.

"Why do you hate me?" I scream. "Why are you keeping me from the only thing in my life that matters?"

Without saying a word, Dad leaves the room.

"Your father can't talk about this right now," Mom says quietly. "He's too angry."

"What's going on? Something's wrong."

Mom takes a deep breath. "Sit down, Kelsi."

My stomach does flip-flops as I sit down next to my mother. She's quiet for a minute. "There are rumors going around town."

"And? What does that have to do with me?"

"They involve your coach."

"What did he do?"

Mom sighs heavily and tucks a strand of wavy blonde hair behind her ear. "Kelsi, your coach is having a relationship with your training partner."

It feels like I've been punched in the stomach. "So? He has a relationship with me too."

"An adult relationship, Kelsi."

"You mean he had sex with her?"

Mom lets out a deep sigh and nods.

"Gross. That can't be true. She's fourteen!"

"I'm sorry, Kelsi. It is true."

"You just said it's a rumor. He's the one person in the world that I trust with my life and my whole, entire future."

47

"I know he's your idol, but a lot of things are starting to make sense all of a sudden, with his behavior. You're too young to understand, but just know that your father and I are making this decision to keep you safe."

I push my chair away from the table and yell, "It's not true. This is bullshit!"

"Kelsi, we're doing this to protect you. You can train elsewhere."

"I don't want to train somewhere else! He's ruined everything for me. I'll never trust anyone again."

Fall 2008

It's our final training exercise, and I'm completely exhausted. Showering and sleeping are luxuries here, and the temperature sends chills through my bones. I'm dressed in my full winter kit, and I'm like a human marshmallow.

Sergeant barks orders as we're each given five live rounds before our next mock operation, or "op," starts. "This is as real as it gets before you go to war. Always remember that right now in Afghanistan, members of the Taliban are coming up with new ways to kill you."

Despite the cold, I feel myself start to sweat as the sergeant continues. "The other units have live rounds too. Fire in one direction so you don't accidentally kill each other. Your goal is to hit them, not us."

He marches down the line and stops in front of me. "Always be one step ahead of the enemy. Think like them and anticipate what they're doing, just like we did with that IED earlier. Don't give the enemy the benefit of the doubt ever. They *will* kill you if you don't kill them first."

He runs his finger down the row. "Remember, the life of your entire unit is in your hands. If one person messes up, someone could actually die."

It's the first true test of how we will cope overseas, and it is intense.

Griffins fly overhead, shooting live rounds out the side doors. Hot brass falls all over us, and smoke bombs are going off everywhere.

Live armored rounds scream through the air. The order comes: "RUN!"

Smoke hangs so heavy in the air that I can barely see in front of me, and the smell of gunpowder swirls in my nostrils. The live fire is loud enough that I can't think, and I'm completely disoriented. In Afghanistan, the enemy will be shooting at us and trying to blow us up with IEDs from underfoot. Will there be any place at all that's safe?

I follow my unit, moving when they move, stopping when they stop, running when they run, and we work together so we don't die, dodging bullets as we race along the frozen Alberta ground. The only thing that makes us remember we aren't actually in Afghanistan is the fact that we can see our breath.

FEAR

```
Is that what I smell?

Are you afraid?

You think it's disorienting now?

Ha, ha, ha. Just you wait.

You're not cut out for war.

Did you ever really think you could do something
like this?

Look at yourself.

You're a child.

The guns are bigger than you are.

Nobody is EVER going to take you seriously.

And that makes them smarter than you.
```

Texas, January 2009

Sweat drops into my eyes. It's so hot out here in the middle of the Texas desert.

For the most part, this landscape is the same as what we will see in Afghanistan. The sun is blisteringly hot, spreading across the wide-open spaces, and I wonder where we will take cover from the enemy. I close my eyes and imagine myself there. I've learned about the vile, heartless things the Taliban do to innocent women, children, and civilians. The mere thought of them puts a sour taste in my mouth and makes me want to go there right now and fight to bring peace to that country.

The climate here is similar to where we're deploying, and I want to figure out how to cope in the hot sun and arid desert. My mouth is dry, my throat is parched, and the six to seven liters of water a day that I'm drinking never seems like enough. We're out here on the range for days at a time, like we could be in Afghanistan, and I'm told even the muted colors of this base are the same as we'll see there.

Hearing movement, I scan the ground. As a person who has to squat to pee outdoors, the fact that poisonous snakes roam freely here and can literally bite you in the ass is rather terrifying. In my imagination, snakes have been slithering up into my bunk bed, hiding in my sleeping bag, and I'm now more afraid of snakes than of the Taliban.

Despite the snakes, overall I'm enjoying this training in Texas because we get to fire the big guns. Shooting ranges are a great way to burn off steam, and there's something delightful about the deafening *boom* of a 155mm round sailing out of an M777 through the air and cracking like thunder over the canyons. It's thrilling to have so much power at my fingertips, especially when after a minute or two we hear, "Target confirmed. Successful hit."

So satisfying.

Each gun troop has two guns at all times—there is never one alone, so it makes for fun competition during the exercise. We each have to get ten rounds down the range, so we make it a race. Both units have unloaded ten rounds and prepped all the fuses to make sure we'll be as quick as possible. Once everyone is in position, we wait for the call.

"Fire mission!" comes over the speaker, and it's go time.

We race to our positions on the guns, with me on the breach. Our first round flies downrange, but our troop is falling behind. My ears ring and I can't hear a thing, rounds fly, the ground shakes, and I'm loving every minute of it, watching this machine toss hundred-pound rounds of ammunition around like toothpicks. Thankfully, we're catching up.

Regardless of the damage this gun can do, I love its sheer force. I don't let myself think too much about who it could be landing on when we're in Afghanistan, but we're being trained to hit targets, not people. And our job as artillery is to protect our infantry that are on dangerous missions outside of the wire. Protecting my fellow soldiers is always most important to me.

We finish the fire mission, pack it in, and head back to base for chow. We barrel for the food line, but then there's an announcement: "Everyone must wash their hands before and after dinner, because people are ill with gastro."

We abandon our trays and head to the washroom, muttering about the news.

"Gastroenteritis." One of the women holds open the door.

"So, stomach flu?"

"Worse. Happened a while back. Someone was sick, didn't wash their hands, and infectious diarrhea spread through the entire base."

Appetizing.

When the taps are turned on, there's no running water. "How the hell is this even allowed?"

She leans over to me. "Welcome to the U.S. military, where we barely get paid, and we don't get clean running water either!"

"Sorry."

I feel bad for her. Apparently, this is the norm for her. We have it good in Canada.

Quebec, January 2009

My eyelids flutter open and adjust to the bright light. I move my hand along my arm to scratch an itch, and my fingers land on a needle. The wrenching pain in my stomach is agonizing, and my eyes follow the line to the IV and watch the drip. How did I get here?

When I hear the familiar voices of Bine and Jen in the distance, I call out weakly, "What's going on?"

"You caught that gastro bug that was going around the base in Texas, Kels," Bine says.

The doctor lays down his chart. "We're admitting you for a couple of days. You're severely dehydrated."

No. I turn to the doctor. "Next week I fly to Cuba with the rest of my unit before our deployment."

"You'll be on IV for at least a couple of days." Jen translates. "Let's worry about getting you healthy before we think about Cuba."

On my third day, I feel well enough to shower and manage to keep down some clear broth. Now that I'm not quite as tired, I'm bored and realize nobody has come to see me since I was admitted. I check my phone and feel a surge in my belly that is not the flu when I see that Brady messaged me: *Haven't heard from you in a while. Everything ok?* It feels good to be thought of. I type back a message: *I died from stomach flu. Was nice knowing you.*

That same afternoon, my sergeant and warrant officer walk into my room, startling me. I sit up in bed and prop myself up on my pillows. "What the hell happened to you, Burns?" Sergeant demands.

"No one told you?"

"Your friends told us when we asked if anyone had heard from you, but you're supposed to let us know where you are at all times." I never thought to check in with anyone at the regiment. I'm basically AWOL!

"It's a severe stomach flu. I've been on IV for almost a week."

"That's why you haven't been to work? You have the flu?"

"I have infectious diarrhea, I'm contagious, and I can't leave until I'm told to leave."

"Follow doctor's orders, Burns." Suddenly he isn't so angry that I haven't shown up for work.

FAMILY

> How does it feel knowing that nobody cares about you?
>
> Remember that day at the recruitment center when you were told that joining the army would help you to form friendships and bonds with the people you serve with?
>
> I can't believe you fell for that.
>
> You're just a number. Nothing more.

FIVE

Sink or Swim

March 2009

The waves bash into the sides of the pier and drench me. I snap one more photo and then wipe off the salt water, stepping away from the pier and the ocean's edge. This is the last picture I wanted to take of this trip. Cuba is gorgeous and has been a dream. I always wanted to get out of my small town and see the world, and the next destination will be Afghanistan. I can't wait.

My foot almost slips on the cold, slippery concrete, and I walk slowly toward the beach. After surviving a gastro infection, I don't need a twisted ankle to prevent me from deploying.

As I move my foot, a massive wave hits me from behind, knocks the wind out of me, and throws me into the water. I hold on to my camera and glasses, then cover my head while the surf tosses me back and forth, sucks me down, and pushes me back up.

The ocean bounces me around like a piece of driftwood, and I claw my way toward the pier. I may be small, but I'm a fighter, and I roll with each surge to gain momentum and work with its force. With every stroke, I'm closer to where I fell in; but just as I'm in range, I get hemmed in between some rocks and have to push off.

A wave grabs ahold of me and tugs me under. I try to steal a breath whenever I surface, but I pull in more water than air. Every fight to the top leads me to another surge that pulls me back under. I'm in big trouble.

My legs grow stiff, and I feel myself sinking down into muted gray-blue. Yes, my life has been tough, but I've always proven stronger, smarter, and braver. I have beaten everyone in basic at their challenges, defied everyone in the unit who had tried to hold me back, and now I'm on my way to war. I just have to get back to the beach, and I can have everything I always wanted. I can't give up.

I kick my legs hard, pushing water out of my lungs as I surface. I dive before a wave takes me under, trying to bob with it, working my way back to shore again. This is where my push-ups and the hours of hard training have come in. I have stamina and endurance, and I can beat this.

From out of nowhere, another wave grabs ahold of me and thrashes me about. All of my efforts drift away as I'm pushed farther from the pier. I never should have come this far out on my own. What was I thinking? But no one wanted to join me. They sat around drinking beer and laughed at me for taking more photos.

I keep swimming against the churning waves, hoping that someone will throw me a lifeline. Someone has to have seen me from shore and called for help by now.

My lungs burn, along with my arms, and dread seeps in. "Help," I call out, but more water gushes into my nose and mouth. Each time a wave pops me up, I grab wildly at the salty air, but nothing holds me.

I'm going to die. I attack the surge just like I fought everything my entire life, but the waves are bigger than me. I start to cough in more water, and suddenly the roar is around me. I see my dad's soft eyes and reach out toward him, but my arm lifts up and bobs in a swell. Why now when I was just starting my own path? I was meant for more than this. My mom's voice pushes through the noise: "Don't quit," and I try to surface, but my legs feel like concrete, and everything becomes a blur.

The next thing I know, I grab on to something solid, and my fingers dig deeper for a hold. My head hurts, and I reach to feel for a bump, but all I touch are thick strands of hair matted with sand. I lick the salt water from my lips, open my eyes, and squint up at the sun. My head turns sharply toward the sound of water, but I'm safe on shore. My shoes are missing, my shirt is ripped, but my camera and glasses are in my hand, and I'm breathing.

Slowly, I sit up, looking in a daze at the calm shoreline, wondering how the hell I came out of the ocean alive without smashing my head on the rocks or slicing myself open on the sharp coral. Never in my life have I faced death. It's the first time I ever felt that level of exhaustion and fear, all elements that might become the norm once I deploy.

I wipe the sand off of my legs and slowly get up. Not a scratch on me, and I know I'm lucky to be alive. My toes wrap around a shell with my first step, and I pick it up as a memento. I turn around for a moment and take one last look at the water lapping at the shore. One of my footprints has almost filled in completely, the other one entirely erased.

Next week when I'm home, I'm going to spend every precious moment with my family. And I'm going to make sure they know how much I love them, in case I don't make it back from my tour. I laugh at the irony of it. This Cuba holiday and my family visit next week is my chance from the military to get my affairs in order in case I don't return from my tour.

* * *

That thought weighs on my mind during the whole week I have with my family, and I spend as much time as I can with them. Everything seems raw somehow, right up until our last evening together.

"Are you sure you don't want us to drive up to see you off?" Dad asks, handing me the placemats.

I look into his eyes, remembering how his face was my last vision before I went unconscious in the ocean, then shift my gaze to the table. I can't help but notice the fading colors of the tattoos on his forearm as he sets the fork next to the plate. I've been soaking in every detail of him, of my home.

"I'm sure."

"We can drive you," Mom pipes in as she pulls a dish from the oven and sets it on the table.

"It's fine, really." I watch the butter melt into the rice, dig out a spoonful, and pass it to Dillon. "We'll say our goodbyes here. It will be easier this way."

"Well, I made your favorite meal for your last evening with us." Mom places a chicken breast on my plate.

"Thanks, Mom. I'll be back before you know it."

Everyone is silent. We've managed to avoid talking about what happens next, and I want to keep it that way. So all through dinner I tell them about some of the funny things during my basic training to keep things light. When the guys taped me up in the cot, how Labonté kept me running with the promise of candy. But it's when Mom clears the table and stands at the edge of the kitchen counter with her shoulders shaking that I know it's on everyone's mind, despite the conversation.

It's my chocolate Lab, Houch, that comes to the rescue, nuzzling my hand as it drops to my side, his tail wagging against the chair. I look into his soft brown eyes. If only everyone could understand like he does.

I roll up the frayed edge of my placemat as Dad says, "It's not like you're just moving away from home or changing schools, kiddo. You're sure you don't want us there?"

I know how I felt when the waves were sucking me under and pounding me against the surf. I wasn't strong enough. What makes me think saying goodbye here will be any easier than tomorrow? I want to tell him that more than anything I would like him and Mom to be there, to give me a hug before I fly to a place where people are trained to kill me. But I can't do it. I need to drive back alone so I can think and put everything in perspective.

"I'm sure, Dad." I walk over and give him a big hug. Part of me wants to stay here forever, with his beard on my neck and the warmth of his body keeping me safe. A bigger part of me, though, wants to go and prove I can do this. This is the career I've chosen, and I've accepted everything that it means. But I'm going to miss them. "Let's go watch some TV," I say, turning away from him so he can't see the tears forming in my eyes.

We go to the couch, where Dillon is already flicking the channels, and we watch a show together. The whole time, Mom and Dad stare at me, like they're trying to memorize my face. For a while Mom rubs my back like she did when I was a little girl, running her fingers through my hair. I feel so helpless in their sadness and lean into Houch's brown fur with a big sigh so they can't hear it. Everything they sacrificed all these years to get enough money for my Tae Kwon Do and nationals tournaments. My tour will likely age them.

When Dillon and Mom go to sleep, Dad gets up from the couch. "Have a beer with me, Kelsi?"

I should be in bed right now, but I find comfort in Dad's voice alone. "Sure."

"I'm hauling a load next week," he says, handing me the bottle.

Houch pads behind him, then settles down with his chin on my knee, his sad brown eyes watching my every move.

"Mom's going with you?"

"Yup."

"That's good."

"Have to take the dog to the vet when we get back."

"Something wrong?"

"He's walking strange. Seems to favor his right leg more. Not unusual for a lab."

I rub Houch's velvety ears. "You better be here when I get back, buddy."

Dad shifts in his chair, and when I look up, his eyes are misty. He starts to say something, but his voice cracks, and instead he takes a swig of beer.

We sit in silence for a long time, then start talking about the weather and sports and things that don't really matter. I want to tell him how I really feel, but that tightness in my chest when I was sinking in the ocean comes right back to me, and my eyes start to tear up.

In the morning, I feel an overwhelming sadness as I lie in bed. Houch pads over to me, and I slide onto the floor and cuddle with him. "I'm going to miss you." I scratch behind his ears. "I can tell you that. I can tell you everything." I lean into his soft fur and hold him until his smooth tongue licks me. I look into his deep brown eyes. "I'm scared, you know that? Scared to leave this all behind, everything that is so good. Am I doing the right thing?"

He whimpers and licks my face.

For the rest of the morning, Houch follows me around wherever I go. When I load my bag in the truck and turn to say goodbye, he's nervously weaving among everyone's legs.

I start with Dillon. I stand on my tip-toes and knock the ball cap off his head. He tosses me around a bit before returning the hat to his head and giving me a long hug. "I love you, sis."

"I love you too."

When I reach for my big, tough dad, he starts crying, and I fight with everything in me to hold back the tears and be strong for him. Houch paws at our legs, whimpering, and Dad pulls back and looks me deep in the eyes and through his tears says, "Love you, kiddo."

Mom is doing her best to keep it together, but when I hug her, I can feel her tears on my shoulder.

When she lets go, she forces a smile, as I do, and we say "I love you" at the same time.

I turn around and step into my truck, wave one last time, and drive away. I look in my rear-view mirror and see Dad and Dillon holding Mom as she sobs. Dillon waves, and I turn the corner.

They're out of sight but not out of mind. I pull over to the side of the road and stare out as if in a fog. My breathing becomes heavy, a mixture of sadness and excitement, fear and wonder. But mostly my family comes back to mind. The next time they see me, I'll no longer be their little girl.

SIX

Home, Sweet Home

March 2009

Water slides through my hair and down my back. I draw a line on the foggy glass door, reach for each drop from the showerhead, each soap bubble that floats into the air. Clean, warm, safe showers aren't waiting for me in Afghanistan as they are here on the base. And definitely not my own private bathroom. I step onto the cold tile floor one foot at a time, savoring each step, every bit of Canada. Facing deployment is weird—everything feels heightened.

My breath quickens as I reach for the hair dryer. I look at myself squarely in the mirror and take some deep breaths to keep my nerves at bay. Leaving for Afghanistan is the moment I've been working toward since I first left home. Most of the night I lay awake, worried that I would sleep through my alarm and miss the flight, but I don't even feel tired! As the heat from the hair dryer flows over my head, I close my eyes and imagine myself in the desert. I'm not sure I should feel so excited that this day is finally here, but my mind is clear, and I am ready to go.

This is the thought I focus on until I'm inside the regiment filled with soldiers saying goodbye. Every time a lump forms in my throat, I remind myself that, for the first time, I feel I'm where I am supposed to be in my life, and it is a beautiful feeling. I'm in the right place. I'm proud to serve my country.

This mantra is harder to hold onto as the room gets more crowded. To my right, an entire family hugs a sobbing mother. Nearby, a soldier kisses a young girl, holding her shaking body. Behind me I hear, "I'll be safe, Dad. I promise."

But right in front of me, a mother strokes her daughter's hair, holding each strand to her face, committing it to memory. I close my eyes and hear Mom say, "You've got this, kiddo," like she has for every single significant event in my entire life. I wish now that I'd asked Mom and Dad to come to see me off, but it's too late. Why did I have to play tough? I would give anything for one of Dad's big bear hugs right now.

I bite my tongue to stop my eyes from welling up and walk slowly toward the medical lineup. This will put me in a different headspace. Last time we got our vaccinations, I almost passed out. I cried, actually, like a small child. Then I remember something from when I was a small child. My mom used to cut out the word "can't" from the dictionary. Anytime I said the word "can't," she would say: "Go get the dictionary. Is that word in there?" I would say: "I can't find it."

It's time to not find my can't.

I brace myself, but before I roll up my sleeve and take a deep breath, the guy jabs me in the back of the arm without *any* warning! I swing my arm forward, causing the needle to fall out.

"Hey! No countdown or anything?"

"Well, now we have to do it again, so I can count if you like."

Ugh!

I sit as still as I can and three, two, one! It burns, but it's over.

AFRAID

> Still afraid of needles?
>
> How do you feel about vicious, murderous religious extremists?
>
> Ah, right.
>
> That's what you signed up for.
>
> The needles were a surprise.
>
> One of these things is going to do much more harm to you than the other.
>
> Can you guess which one?

A day later, it's the first time I'm calling my parents from overseas, and with each number I press, the farther I feel from home. My eyes well up again, and I set down the phone till I can pull myself together. I have three days with the troops before we fly to Kandahar, and the barracks we are in right now is covert, so I can't even tell my parents what country we are in. All I can say is I'm in a stopover place—I have to be tough.

The nine-and-a-half-hour time difference is drastic, and I know my parents won't be awake, but I need to hear a voice from home, even if it is through the answering machine. We hit the ground running tomorrow, and I'm nervous. But I won't tell them that.

I dial again, and my stomach sinks with the silence after each ring. *Pick up. Please.*

A tear starts to roll down my cheek. I just saw them a couple of days ago, but I've never been so far from home.

The answering machine comes on, and I close my eyes at the sound of their voices, wishing them right here with me. The beep comes all too soon. "Hi guys, it's me. We made it here safe. Guess what? We had the whole plane to ourselves." I grit my teeth, then continue rambling on in my usual style. "The heat is so intense, it's like someone's holding a blow dryer over my head, and has it on full blast. I'll call tomorrow if I can. Love you."

When I get back to my room, I label and categorize my clothes and boots as a distraction. It's more like a dorm with bunk beds than a hotel, but it's world-class compared to Farnham. I shower, and a bit of cool water feels incredible. It's the first time I've stopped sweating since being here. After drying off, I am still wet and realize that I will be permanently sweating as long as I'm in this part of the world.

I crawl into my bed with the crazy awareness that tomorrow we go to war. My alarm is set for 0500, but I won't need it. Everything seemed so far away yesterday, but now it's sinking in that I'm actually here. I don't expect I'll sleep much tonight.

It was a little over two years ago that I chose this amazing career, and it has already taken me so far. I've been all over Canada, through the U.S., Cuba, and now I'm heading to Kandahar.

Earlier tonight, I was eating ice cream with a bunch of people I barely know, to whom I'll soon be trusting my life in a war zone in Afghanistan. I didn't make the close bonds during BMQ that I was promised the day I signed up for the forces, but I'm sure now that once we're in the field it will come together. I saw during our mock battles that when we're in the thick of it, soldiers have each other's backs.

My chest tightens at the thought of war, and I close my eyes and burrow into the starched sheets; I really need to try and sleep.

I shift on my pillow and look at my watch: 0300. In a couple hours, the Hercules transport plane will take us from our stopover place to Afghanistan, and we've been briefed on what to expect. Joining me on that beast of a plane will be a whole battery of artillery soldiers. The flight will take five hours, and during the last hour, when we head into Afghan airspace, we have to put our kit on, since that's when things become dangerous. I'm excited to get out there and put my skills to the test for the next six months.

I take a deep breath and think of my new lover. Its name is mangosteen. A lot of the local food is not exactly up my alley (camel milk is *not* my thing), but these juicy, white, fleshy fruits are incredible, and I can't get enough of them. Wish I had some now to quiet my mind enough so I could get to sleep. Even more, I wish Mom were here to rub my back like she did when I was little.

0400. In a few hours, I will hand over my civilian clothes, which I won't need until our next leave or at the end of our tour. Then I'll make my way in line for my plates, vests, weapons, ammo, helmet, and webbing. Our gear was shipped over months ago while I was still training back in Canada. Now I have to sign for it all, because it's mine for now, and I'm responsible for anything that goes missing on our ops. I am happy and nervous all at the same time. I try not to think about the soldier who had this kit before me and why it wasn't needed anymore.

My alarm goes off at 0500, and I bolt out of bed to pack up my things. I chuckle to myself, thinking about how everything is jammed in my bag right now, when back in basic everything had to be folded so perfectly! I remember one of the officers telling me once, "Calm down, Burns, it's just a game." Soon I'll find out if that was true.

I lace up my boots, custom-made for me because my feet are so small. Small but mighty. That's me. But I'm ready for war. Here we go.

WELCOME

Kelsi, finally you've made it to *war*.

I've been *waiting* for so long.

Right now, you think you're "small but mighty," but you're so *wrong*.

You're small, yes.

But *mighty*? Ha.

You're anything but.

SEVEN

Afghanistan

April 2009

My stomach reels as the plane flies in tactical motion, in case someone tries to shoot us down. I'm pulled back, squeezing the bottom of my seat as we accelerate quickly and then drop.

I lurch forward. We zoom up again, then side-to-side, then down. I might throw up, but it's so much fun.

The new normal is that people don't like us here. But then again, I've been bullied for my entire life; this time, though, the bullies happen to have access to explosives.

We make it to Kandahar and to the Kandahar Air Force (KAF) base. This base is a large "safe" area where NATO runs everything in and out of Afghanistan. The division of the Canadian Army I'm in is under NATO. In fact, this base is where more than thirty-six countries are working together to bring down the Taliban and restore peace for the civilians. And now I'm a part of this meaningful mission—to help the innocent Afghan people.

The door of the Herc opens, and we all step out. It isn't nearly as humid here as it was where we flew in from. It's a nice, dry, fifty-degree heat, and it's actually quite comfortable. While we unload, others on the tarmac are loading up to leave. They're finished their tour or are heading out for their home leave travel. They look exhausted.

"Bine! Jen!" I spot my friends minutes after getting off the bus. I have never been so happy to see two familiar faces.

"Welcome to KAF." Jen gives me a big hug.

"How are you guys doing?" I wrap my arms around Bine and give her a squeeze. "You've been here a week now?"

"Yes. Waiting to get briefed to find out where we're going. We're sharing a room. You should stay with us tonight and we can catch up!"

"I can't wait to find out where my guns are waiting for me."

"Let's grab dinner." Bine points to the boardwalk that leads from the Canadian side of KAF to the American side. "There's a Subway here."

"And beach volleyball too!" Jen giggles.

I chuckle at the thought. "How about a shop that sells toothbrushes?"

Dozens of uniformed soldiers stroll along the boardwalk, weapons strapped to their backs, takeout containers in hand. Other soldiers sit at picnic tables, eating Subway and checking their email on laptops. In true Canadian style, there's a group of people playing ball hockey on the regulation-size hockey rink right here in the middle of the desert. It's comforting to have so many reminders of home, and I guess that's why all of this is here.

Home. I spot a place with computers and phones for soldiers to use. "Do you guys mind if I call my folks real quick?"

"No, go ahead."

I go inside and key in my parents' phone number. They're probably working, but it's worth a try.

I let the phone ring, prepared for the machine to answer, but someone picks up. "Mom!"

"Kelsi, we missed your call the other night."

Silence. Is she crying?

"Kiddo," Dad says.

"Hey! I'm at the base now. You should see it. I'm in the middle of the desert and they have a Tim Hortons and a ball hockey rink!"

They're both silent now. Growing up, I got used to Dad being the one to call and check in with us when he was on the road. Now the tables have turned, but I treasure the sound of his voice even more now than I did back then.

"Dillon says to say hi," Dad blurts out.

"And Nana," adds Mom.

Silence again. Am I the one that's going to cry now?

"Thanks. I love you both," I stammer. "And don't worry about me." Ridiculous. Of course they'll be worrying about their nineteen-year-old daughter going to war.

"Be careful, kiddo. Keep your eyes open." Dad's voice is quieter than usual.

"I love you guys." I manage to get that out without choking up.

MORE TIME

Ah.

You should have talked to them a little bit longer, Kelsi.

So you could leave them with more of the old you.

The you they said goodbye to when you left for Afghanistan.

The you that they will never see again.

Oh, well.

Too late!

"Afghanistan is a big sandbox with bombs hidden everywhere." Sergeant lifts up a cigarette box to demonstrate. "This can take your legs off." He points to a big barrel. "That one can blow you up while you're inside a tank."

He looks each of us in the eye. "IEDs come in every size and can do a wide range of damage."

IED training is a wake-up call. There are vehicle-borne IEDs (VBIEDs) and even donkey-borne IEDs (DBIEDs). The types of IEDs include centralized, daisy-chain, pressure-plate, secondary-device, remote-detonated, and the good old-fashioned land mine.

"There's scary shit waiting for you outside the wire." Sergeant motions us farther into the fenced-in area of KAF. "The Taliban is made up of very smart, resourceful people. They'll use anything they can get their hands on to make IEDs. Something that looks like a discarded cigarette package or a piece of garbage can be an explosive."

Thank God for this briefing. If I have to go outside the FOB (forward operating base) without my artillery unit, I will likely be on foot, so I need to know what I might be up against and understand as much as I can.

He motions to objects lying on the ground. "Tell me which ones are the IEDs. And treat it as if these are explosives. Move cautiously."

We balance our weight, pointing out items that meet his nod of approval. He walks around, highlighting items so everyone is aware.

"The Taliban are crafty. They're always watching, and they're always listening. They know we use metal detectors to find their bombs in the ground before we step or drive over them. They change shit up." He picks up what looks like a piece of trash from the ground and holds it up to our faces. "They're using less metals that can be detected in the ground. Now they're using plastic for the outer shell of their bombs. You need to get good at spotting anything that doesn't quite belong."

So, basically, I can't walk by anything that looks like litter. An IED can be anywhere and anything.

EVERYWHERE

This IED training will stay in your brain forever, Kelsi.

You won't have to work to recall it.

It will become part of you.

Every single time you walk down a city street, litter equals possible death.

It will bond us.

Well, unless the training fails you and you blow yourself up, of course.

Nothing to get yourself too worked up about.

EIGHT

FOB Ramrod

April 2009

I stare at the door gunners hanging off the back tail of the Chinook as we fly away from KAF. There are two more gunners up by the pilots. Never in my wildest dreams would I have imagined this is where I'd be at nineteen years old. I'm seated in the belly of a flying whale, zooming across a war zone, with roughly thirty other soldiers. Nobody speaks, because the Chinook is deafening. My stomach is in knots, yet I can't stop smiling. I've never felt so alive. I've been addicted to adrenaline for as long as I've known how to feel. It's part of my genetic makeup.

We're on our way to a U.S. forward operating base (FOB), "Ramrod," where we'll be until the end of this tour. We'll be the only Canadians there, and most of my unit can't speak English. I'll be one of the people helping us communicate with the Americans; besides the officers who are multilingual, they'll be able to understand me.

We'll only be back at KAF if something bad happens, until it's our turn for our home leave travel, or if we die. Another fun new reality—the chances of everyone in this Chinook returning in one piece are pretty slim. I'm okay with that. I know what I signed up for.

The land below shows greener than I ever expected, even though it seems pretty dry and dusty for the most part. We've been flying for a while, and the landscape continues to spread out before me. In the distance, mountains edge the horizon, and the compounds are tiny specks. Those are the homes that harbor the enemy we're looking for.

From this vantage point, they look so small and inconsequential with their mud walls and thin roofs, but you never know who lives inside of them. FOB Ramrod is farther from KAF than I thought, and an even greater distance from Canada.

The farther away I am, the more I miss home. It's the little things, like riding dirt bikes with Dillon, seeing Dad off as he turns from the driveway, and smelling Mom's cooking.

The Chinook lands in the middle of a field inside the FOB. It's so small you can see the buildings and tents lined up from one end of it to the other. The property I grew up on had more acreage than this! Not a lot of space, but we're told there's a chance we'll be working with the Americans and doing a lot of shooting. Working more means missing home less, and I need to keep myself distracted. Besides, I'm looking forward to doing the job I was sent here to do.

When we deplane, a sweltering, over one hundred degree heat hits us. We unload our gear with dust swirling at our feet and carry our kits and the one box each of us was allowed to bring over here. Mine is mostly filled with soap, shampoo, and other toiletries. We trudge with our kits down to one side of the FOB, where there are two beautiful M777 howitzers facing south, just waiting to be fired. Before that can happen, though, I need to make my way to our tent.

We're coming in after a reserve artillery unit from Canada, and they had five tents set up. One of them is for the officers, one for the sergeant and warrant officer, one to serve as a kitchen and sitting area with TV and snacks, one for radio communications, and then one for our unit.

A Canadian flag flies above our tent, and at the very front entrance there's a little coffee breakfast area among more dust and dirt. At the overhang of the tent is a noose, and we're not sure if it's meant to make us laugh or feel uncomfortable, but it does both. One of the guys takes it down. A little too sinister.

Walking into the tent, I'm excited to see that the people here before us made separation walls, giving each of us a little private area of about 7 x 7. There's a cot in each one, and I claim the best "room" of all, which must have been set up by a woodworker. My walls are cut out of plywood to make it look like I'm in a castle. I have shelves for my socks, a custom wooden dowel for hanging my kit, a spot for my boots, and the best part? A coffee table perfect for sitting with a laptop or to set a fan on.

The final touch is a beautiful carving sitting there—a hand-carved artillery M777 howitzer shooting a round downrange into the table. Whoever was here before me made a little room inside of a tent feel like home.

Afghanistan, however, is anything but home. On my first fire watch shift, I cringe at a spider the size of a dinner plate creeping up the wall. "What the hell is that?"

"Camel spider," my partner says matter-of-factly. "Chews on you while you sleep."

"Yuck."

I squint behind my goggles to focus on my watch: 0228. My partner and I are two and a half hours into our shift. Along with the Americans that have their tower on the other side, our unit is here to provide cover fire for the Americans and another unit on op about thirty kilometers away. We can be called for a fire mission at any time. I'm on edge, but I'm ready.

"RADIO CHECK, OVER," I respond to the main radio controller.

Other than radio checks every half hour, my partner and I chat to keep each other awake as we watch. We converse in French, since he doesn't speak English, but we talk about nothing, really.

"Can you believe we're actually here?"

"No, it's crazy, isn't it?"

Once we finally received our night-vision goggles (NVGs), I can see everything clearly now, the only difference is the color—it's green. I can see into a compound with no roof a little distance ahead. There's a family inside with a few small children, some sheep, and cows.

"Do sheep ever sleep?"

"Dunno."

Silence.

"Did you hear that?" he asks.

My blood runs cold. Is there something in the brush? I cock my head to listen.

"Nothing besides that gunfire off in the distance."

"Must have been an animal."

I look back into the compound, watching one of the children stirring in their sleep. It freaks me out that I'm being watched right this very second as well. We know the Taliban is outside these walls, and I cling to my rifle. It's not a question of whether they will attack, but when. If we did take fire, it would make the night go by faster, but is that really what I want?

Just before our shift ends, a frail girl skips barefoot out of her compound, leading a cow down a dusty path. She seems to be singing to herself, her long brown hair swinging over her bony shoulders. She stops for a moment, looks up at the tower, and then lifts her long fingers and waves at me.

I wave back, and a big smile flashes across her round face.

"Emma," I whisper. The nickname makes her more real to me. As she continues down the path, her innocent face is still before me, a reminder of why I'm here fighting the Taliban—so she doesn't have to grow up under their oppressive regime.

* * *

Every day for the past month has been pretty much the same routine under an unrelenting sun. We haven't seen much action here on the guns, but it's a powerful feeling when we get to blow stuff up.

Tents shake and rattle, and the ground moves beneath our feet when we fire explosives downrange to help a unit outside the FOB. We never ask where it's landing, but we hit the target. The Americans sit on top of their tanks and cheer when we blast the enemy.

The best is when we receive fire mission orders early in the morning when everyone is still sleeping. We start blasting rounds downrange and watch the Americans run out of their tent, not knowing what the hell is happening.

My other routine is hitting the gym tent with Sergeant Leblond, where we talk guns and strength. It's basically a canopy with camouflage netting down the sides, covering barbells, free weights, and some kettlebells.

"Ten more, away, let's go Burns," barks Leblond, his round face glistening with sweat.

"Then we're done?"

"Or you can do a few laps around the running track."

My arms are burning, but I drop to the bench for another set of hanging triceps dips. Since I got here, he's been helping condition me so that I'll be strong enough to handle the heavy rounds of ammo. He's making sure there'll be no reason for the guys in my unit to say I'm not capable. The most important thing to me is that they know I can keep up with them. Given my size, I always feel like I have something to prove, so I make sure that I carry my weight and work just as hard as they do. Because someday I hope to lead them. I like to lead. I don't want to follow anyone. In order to be a leader like Leblond, you've got to be damn well good at it. When I get good enough, I'll become the leader.

After I do a few cooldown stretches on the mats, I pick up my bag.

"What's your hurry?"

"Laundry."

By the time I reach the end of the dusty path to the laundry tent, a fresh-faced American named Gould is waiting on the wooden steps to the tent.

"Got it?"

I nod and hand him my laptop while I dump my clothes into the machine.

He's looking at a photo and then shoves it in his pocket.

"Your girlfriend?" I ask.

He nods. "You?"

"There's a guy back home that I'm into, but it's casual. At least till I get back home."

"Sexting, eh?"

We both laugh. I've made friends with lots of the Americans here. Many of the Americans haven't worked with women because of their male-dominated trades, and they appreciate how I take their shit and give it right back. It lets them see me as an equal soldier and helps me to earn their trust. Ultimately, by joking around with me, they're showing that I have their respect, and that means the world to me.

I'm still finding sand in my braid from the storm yesterday. It was like fine dust, but it pelted my face and seeped into my tent and my hair.

"I can't believe you used buckets and a washing board before you got to use the American machines," Gould teases.

"It's just training if we need to go outside the wire."

"I know, but it's pioneer-like."

I jab him in the arm. "Remember, the Canadians have the Internet."

"But we have the best gear."

"And we have the soft drinks."

"What do you care? You're always drinking water." A sly smile rises from his square jaw.

"We're in the desert, for Christ's sake!"

He leans against the machine. "I would give anything for a Coke right now."

"No wonder you guys are banned from drinking soda," I chuckle. "Dehydration isn't funny, Gould." I can't imagine not drinking water here. It's so refreshing.

"I still want a Coke so bad."

"How many cans of Coke for a pair of Oakleys?" I pull a can from my pack.

He peers over his sunglasses, the dark frames sliding down his long nose. "How many pairs do you want?"

"Just one." I hand him two cans of soda, and he passes over his sunglasses. "For real?"

He cracks open the Coke with a wide smile. "For real."

We sit down on the steps while dust swirls around our feet. Gould hits "play" on the Dane Cook comedy album on my laptop for our weekly laundry ritual, and we laugh until the wash is done.

* * *

I'm awakened from a dead sleep at 0530 by mortar rounds, handguns, and rifles ringing out and going off everywhere. My heart pounds as I jump to my feet, grab my weapon, and run outside. We must be under attack, maybe even overrun. I race to my plates and helmet with everyone else. We grab our guns, suit up, and wait for the fire mission call. I hear screaming in a language I hadn't heard much and realize it's coming from the Afghan workers who sleep outside the FOB for protection from the Taliban.

We're ready with the big guns and mortars.

"False alarm!" the sergeant yells, and we duck under the cover of a tent as shrapnel rains down in tiny pieces.

"What the hell happened?" I ask Bless, Gould, and McMillin as we're lined up at the chow hall, where both groups, Canadian and American, eat together.

Gould chuckles. "Someone dropped a mortar round inside the shipping container that holds our confiscated ammunition and IED parts."

"Jesus, we're lucky nobody was hurt."

"Very." McMillin dimples deepen as he smiles. "That soldier will be sent back to KAF."

The Army doesn't particularly appreciate you almost killing a bunch of your own people, even if it is an accident. Each person is responsible for their actions, and it's not often we get a second chance. I am fine with the responsible person leaving.

We grab our trays, scoop our breakfast, and sit down at big bench tables with Bless and a few of the other guys.

"I'll get you an extra mango passion fruit popsicle and trade it for a Coke," says Gould.

"You're on!"

McMillin is about a foot taller than Gould, but they're close like brothers and have been on a couple tours together. They're infantry and know what it's like outside the wire. I love listening to their stories, since I probably won't find out what it's like first-hand, being artillery.

A heavily tattooed American joins us where we're sitting. "Have you been outside the wire yet?" he asks me.

"No."

"A lot of it you don't want to see." This guy has a line tattooed on the back of his neck, along with the words *Cut here*, which sums up his sense of humor.

"Careful, these stories aren't appropriate for her," Gould jokes.

"Hey! I want to hear."

"Like about women being stoned to death for looking at a man."

"You've actually seen it happen?"

"Yes. Not far away from here. They bury the women up to their necks and throw rocks at them until they die."

"Jesus."

I graduated from high school two years ago, but here I'm getting a different kind of education. So many people are victims of the Taliban, and that's one of the reasons I'm here is to help them.

Gould motions to a guy at the next table. "He's one of the humanitarians here and goes into villages to help people."

"We go in to shoot them down."

"But you can't think about that. Our job is different than theirs. We're working together."

"Either way, Burns. It's not pleasant out there." Bless raises his bushy eyebrows. "If you ever end up outside, don't volunteer for shit."

"He's right," says Gould. "Don't be a hero. Just do your job and come back. I can't lose my Coke dealer."

HURT

You hurt for these people?

Since when?

Where are those bombs landing?

You're not exactly an innocent player here, Kelsi.

You have an awful lot of blood on your hands…

NINE

Invisible Enemy

"Burns, you're on GD today!" ribs McMillin as he and Gould join me on general duty on the American side of the FOB.

"Yeah, thrilling." I love these guys, and they're making being on tour that much easier.

"Hey, Burns, you speak French, right?"

"*Oui*, Gould."

"Why don't you talk to many of the other Canadians?"

I look over at a group of guys from my unit on the other side of the yard who are loudly conversing in French, then back to Gould. "Ever see them talking to me?"

"Not really."

"That's why."

"What's wrong with them?" McMillin asks, glaring at them over his sunglasses.

I take a deep sigh. "Some thought it's because I didn't party with them back in Quebec, or because I beat them at physical stuff. I just don't really care to get to know them any better at this point. We have each other's backs on the guns, but I don't need friends like that."

"Their loss," Gould shrugs.

I am grateful for the relationships I'm building with them. I'm beginning to feel accepted, which helps, because I don't feel that from my own unit. I've always craved the structure of a group, even when being betrayed by that very structure when I'm trying my hardest.

"So, is watching Afghan workers build concrete pads your thing, Burns?" Bless joins us, his square shoulders blocking the sun.

"After what you guys told me yesterday, I like them a lot less than before."

Gould kicks at the dust. "Wait till they blow up your buddy with an IED. You never know when one of them can be a Taliban plant. I don't trust any of them."

McMillin adjusts his gun. "Or rolling in a Hummer, taking fire from the rooftops, not knowing where in the city the enemy is hiding among a crowd of civilians. We've lost a lot of guys to them."

"We've lost friends," says Bless.

"I've only been here a few weeks, but I'm happy that in Canada our tours are six months. How do you guys handle one year?"

Gould smirks. "Lots of soda."

We all laugh. Many of the Americans have already done tours in Afghanistan and Iraq. Some are on their first tour, like me, but others are on their third or fourth. I don't know how they can be away for so long. Afghanistan isn't a new war for Canada, but until 2007, we'd been doing UN missions rather than combat, so our role here is pretty new.

The guys turn their attention to an Afghan worker, and Gould reminds me, "Even though the workers are screened, be on your guard. I don't trust any of them."

With that, I tilt my tan hat to shield some of the sun, but it's impossible—the rays still bounce off the sand and come at me from every angle.

As Gould walks away, one of the Afghan workers approaches me and complains, "I am not feeling well." I'm surprised at how good his English is. "Can I have Gatorade?"

"You know where the cooler is," I tell him, pointing to the fridge the workers use. I'm hot, thirsty, and have little patience for Afghan men in general, especially after the things I've heard.

"Can you show me?" he asks through his thick beard.

I start walking closer to the cooler, and he stops me. "You're new here? How many Canadians are here?"

I scrutinize him carefully, the long pants and shirt, the hand-stitched hat with beading on it. It's true the majority of Afghan people are innocent, including these guys who are working for us infidels to provide for their families, but I can't trust any of them.

The trouble is, everyone is dressed in civilian clothes, so the enemy is invisible to us, and danger is everywhere. Every burka, every turban, every person who looks like this man is the enemy in my mind, including these "screened" Afghan workers. I have to assume they all want to kill me. My life depends on that judgment.

"You know you aren't supposed to be talking to me."

"The others don't speak English. When is your shift over?" I am very aware of my rifle right now. "Are those guns new? When did they come in?"

"None of your business."

"Why are they pointing that way?"

"You know you can't ask those questions."

"Oh no, I'm sorry," he says and goes off back to work.

I don't like this guy, so I keep my eye on him. In a few minutes, he's coming back up to me. "Those are very big guns. How far can they shoot?"

"Yeah, they are big, and it's none of your business."

"Can they be moved? Where is the ammunition? I don't see it."

"Go!"

He walks away.

One of the Americans has heard the conversation. He leans over to me and says quietly, "Put a round in the chamber and stay ready."

Holy shit, what just happened?

Gould notices and is by my side as the American jogs away and comes back two minutes later. He's barreling toward us on a gator, his face covered with a bandana, and a bunch of US Army guys in civilian clothes with big beards and masks are with him.

They jump out of the rig with rifles raised and begin hollering at the Afghan guy.

The other Afghan workers run toward us with their hands up, shouting in Farsi, waving their arms around in big, animated gestures.

The other soldiers dash over and point their rifles at the workers. "Get back to work!"

The American grabs the man who was asking me too many questions. He looks at me, crying, "Miss! Miss! No! What did I do? Ma'am, what did I do?"

"You know you aren't supposed to be asking those kinds of questions," I yell back at him.

"No, ma'am, please. What did I say?" He's crying now, and as hard as I try, I can't help but feel a bit sorry for him when I see the fear in his eyes.

One of the Americans screams in his face. "You shut the *fuck* up and you don't talk to her. Don't look at her. Face forward."

He starts begging, "No! I didn't know! I'm sorry, I didn't know!"

They push the man to the ground on his knees and zip-tie his hands behind his back. A part of me worries that I may have overreacted.

"No, Miss! No, Miss! I didn't do! I didn't do!"

They tug a blindfold over his eyes while he screams and cries, "Where am I going, ma'am?! Please!"

The guys keep bellowing, "Shut the fuck up!"

I can't answer him. I'm done. I don't know where he's going, but I'm pretty sure he won't be coming back.

They throw the weeping man in the back of the gator, and the guys in civilian clothes and masks take him away. I assume he will be interrogated for the rest of the day.

I look from side to side. Did that really just happen? I wonder what they're doing to him.

Gould turns to me, "You okay?"

I nod.

"Remember," he sips from the can. "Don't give anyone the benefit of the doubt. They won't give it to you."

I pull my rifle a little tighter as I continue watching the rest of the workers build, like nothing ever happened.

Later, at our side of the FOB, Sergeant Leblond approaches me.

"Burns, I hear you were involved in an incident today with one of the Afghan workers?"

"Yes." I feel a knot in my stomach. "Did I do something wrong?"

He shakes his head. "That man did not have ID or security clearance to be working inside the FOB. He was planted by the Taliban to gather intelligence."

"Shit, how did that happen?"

"I don't know." He looks down, then back at me. "You know they have little respect for women, so he probably thought you would be dumb enough to tell him anything he wanted to know. There's a reason we've been trained to hate them. You did good, Burns."

I shift my weight. "The Taliban was right there, in plain clothes. Someone even the military thought was a civilian."

He nods. "This is war. All the rules of behavior are off the books. You're darker-skinned, you're the enemy. All our lives here depend on that judgment."

I head back to my tent and continue processing this information. I came face-to-face with the enemy. The taste of bile rises in my throat.

ENEMY

Remember his face.

You'll be seeing it again.

Well, likely not in person.

But you'll see men like him in your dreams.

And in every airport and shopping mall and grocery store you ever enter again for the rest of your sad little life.

TEN

"Borrowed"

I'm still rattled when I get back to the Canadian side of the FOB. I want to have a shower, some snacks, and watch TV; but as soon as I get in, one of the guys tells me, "Burns, *Sergent veut te voir dans la tente radio.*"

Why would the sergeant want to see me in the radio tent? I work on the guns, not in communications.

I walk into the tent and quickly find the sergeant. "You wanted to see me, Sergeant Leblond?"

He doesn't look pleased. "Yes. I just got a call. Come with me."

He walks me over to a bunch of maps that are laid out on a table.

"Look, Burns. You're going out on an operation soon."

"What? But we don't move guns."

"This has nothing to do with the guns. You're being borrowed by the Brits."

"I don't understand."

"You're being tasked to go with a British infantry unit next week on a foot operation outside the wire."

My heart is racing. "The British? Whoa. Why me?"

"They need a female solider to search women and children, and you've been selected to go."

Yes! It's go time. I'm getting the chance to do the job I wanted from the very beginning.

My sergeant doesn't look as happy. His eyebrows are drawn together on his bald head, and his strong jaw is set. "Listen, I'll be honest with you, Burns. I'm not happy to take you off the guns, because it leaves us short-handed, but I also know what you're walking into. I've tried to convince them to take someone else."

I want to say, *Why are you trying to hold me back?*

"With all due respect, Sergeant, I wanted to be infantry from the very beginning. I chose guns because they said I'd be too small to do infantry. I want to do it."

"The Brits are heavy hitters. They're all over and have a reputation for being ruthless and tough."

"I know the Brits. I can handle it."

He tilts his head and looks at me. "

"Regardless of how either of us feels about it, it's come down the chain of command, and you're going."

"I'll be fine! I feel like you've prepared me, and I am willing to go."

"Don't kid yourself. Nobody can prepare you for what you'll see out there, Burns."

To the best of his ability, and with the little information he has, he starts pointing out spots on the maps where I will be going. "Since the British occupy a different area than the Americans and Canadians, you'll be in a place you've not been briefed on. It's one of the most dangerous areas in Afghanistan, known as the birthplace of the Taliban." He continues. "When you get back to KAF, you'll be picked up by the British, brought over to their side of the base, and given a full breakdown of what you'll be doing, for how long, and why. You'll meet with the Canadian military police to be given some gloves, learn the proper searching techniques, and what you're going to be looking for during your searches. It will be brief but will give you more of an idea of what you'll be doing outside the wire."

"All right."

"It's important that you understand that as a searcher, even though you'll be going to be with the Brits, you'll be making the judgment calls on who and what to search. You are your own boss for the most part on this op. The Brits will tell you which units need you and where, but other than that, your job will be to search any and all of the women and children that you encounter."

I can't quite hide my excitement, and a smile spreads across my face as I leave the radio tent.

* * *

Word has spread to the rest of my artillery unit that I am going outside the wire with the Brits and that I'll be gone for at least a week. Most of the guys are pissed off because I get to do "some cool shit" and also because now they'll be short-handed on the guns and fire watch. They have to pick up the slack for me while I'm gone, and most of them are less than happy with this.

Some of them tell me, "You don't deserve to go," and, "You won't even know what to do once you get out there." I can't wait to get away from them for a while.

On the other hand, Gould and some of the guys are proud. "The Brits have a solid reputation. They're tough."

"Badass," says Gould, and then he teases, "Well, I guess this is a good time for you to get one of those *Cut here* tattoos, in case the Taliban gets ya?"

I laugh. They give me hugs and wish me luck.

Sergeant Leblond takes me to a small range area the Americans have made to make sure I feel 100 percent comfortable with my weapon and kit. We go through drills until I can access everything I need at the drop of a hat. "Remember, keep your eyes open. It's not a game."

He clearly knows more about where I'm going and what I'll be doing than I do. Just like he's helped me at the gym to make sure I'm strong enough to handle the job physically, he's giving me extra support on my weapons training. He takes off some of the tactical gear for his C7 and gives it to me to use. He even strips his C7 bare down to the stock setting and makes my weapon look like something out of a movie. No matter what, he has my back. I am grateful for this man.

"Always watch where you step. Make sure what you're doing, you're doing properly." His French accent is one I'll miss. "Remember, you're in charge of yourself out there. Do your job and don't embarrass us."

Thanks to him, I feel like I can do this, and I know he believes in me. He is doing his best to make sure I can handle myself outside the wire and that I will be able to come back to my unit alive; but as far as I can tell, nobody else in my own unit actually cares if I come back at all.

TRUST

Kelsi, doesn't this man remind you of anyone?

The way he's taken you under his wing.

The way he's given you so much attention and pushes you so hard?

He knows you can succeed.

He makes you believe in yourself.

Remember the last time you idolized a man like this?

Remember how that ended for you? Can you trust him?

There are a few people in the Chinook with me, including some Afghan interpreters, "terps," also heading back to KAF. We lift up, and just like that, we're out of the FOB's safe zone, and the dust ball that follows clouds my vision as we fly over the guns.

Shit. I'm going outside the wire, on foot, in front of the guns. My stomach is in knots with nerves and excitement.

We fly very low the entire way—lower than I've ever flown—and I keep hoping we don't take any rounds. Fortunately, we land in KAF without any issue.

I'm taken to the Canadian side of the base and am read the riot act about how to handle myself with the British. I will be the only Canadian with these guys there, and basically, as Leblond said, I am in charge of myself, searching the women and children we encounter and having the guys' backs once we get out there.

I spend some time with the military police and become familiar with the power of a very versatile invention: zip-ties. They are efficient and strong. I'm coached on how to take someone down and hold them in a fairly uncomfortable position until I'm done searching them and their home for various different "things" they aren't supposed to have.

On the British side of KAF, I'm introduced to a unit I will now be attached to.

"Welcome to Alpha Company," Sergeant Major says as he leads me aside. "You'll be working with our platoon. Stay low and move fast, listen to the NCOs (noncommissioned officers) and platoon sergeants, and all should be fine. Charles!" He motions to a short, stocky guy.

I strain to understand what's being said to me in a thick Scottish accent. I've never worked with a unit from a country besides Canada and the U.S., and I could clearly understand most of them, but wow. The British are a whole new ball game.

"Aye. What ye taking me away from Scoff for?"

"Burns, your female searcher." Sergeant Major steps back and sizes me up. "Don't know what you know, but we are the aviation assault group. Fly in, fuck shit up, fly out. Do not slow us down and don't hesitate to fire. This is Sergeant Charles. You'll be working with him."

Charles looks at me with the kindest eyes. "And always have a battle buddy." He points to the far end of the room. "That tall Fijian is Rav, and the red-haired bloke is Vince. They're the only non-Scottish in the group. Mick next to him is as new as you are. Been with us less than a month. That skinny guy on the other side of him is Max."

"And Johnny!" He calls out to a tall, muscular man across the room and motions him over.

"This is Section Commander Johnny. They're not all built like him. Johnny could bench press a car."

Johnny shifts his weight and pulls his shoulders back proudly. When he opens his mouth, it's also to speak in a Scottish accent. "We'll have a kit check before the next op, so make sure your kit is squared. Make sure you have ten liters of water in your daysack and some warm kit, as the Afghani nights are freezing."

I love listening to these guys talk, but I really have to work to figure out what they're saying.

Johnny stands stiffly till Sergeant Major ribs him. "These guys have been here for a few months, so please do realize they are probably mega horny."

"Oh, you're a right scunner," Johnnys deep-set eyes twinkle.

Sergeant Major laughs and points to a guy with a cigar hanging out the side of his mouth. "That's Watson. He has no game, so you're safe, but stay away from these other guys." He winks.

"Ya plum." Johnny shakes his head.

Sergeant Major slaps Johnny on the shoulder. "They're all good blokes. They've got your back."

Johnny sucks on his cigarette, and his wide chest fires out smoke in deliberate bursts. "They don't have many women and children sticking around where we're headed, so you won't be needed much."

I'm not sure how to feel about that, but we are told to meet outside the tents at 0100 to load on a bus that will deliver us to the landing zone with the Chinook. From there, we will fly to the Panjwai district, one of the most dangerous parts of southern Afghanistan.

Before we board that Chinook, we stand at attention for a ramp ceremony. The sound of bagpipes gives me chills as a casket draped with a Canadian flag is pushed onto the tarmac. Another soldier is being sent home in a box as I prepare to fly deeper into the conflict that claimed his life.

BUCKLE UP

Things are about to get interesting for you, Burns.

You may want to take a moment.

Your life will never be as good as it is right now.

But, of course, you can't know that.

Not yet.

So, good luck!

PS: You really should call your parents one last time.

Don't forget, even if you make it home in one piece, that doesn't mean you'll be okay.

ELEVEN

The Op

We're locked and loaded in a packed Chinook. Sitting on the floor is my only option, and my body vibrates the entire time. We've been flying in the pitch black, and I have no idea where we are, but we've been in the air for hours, so we have to be close. We're given the two-minute warning by Sergeant Charles, his Scottish accent slowly becoming easier for me to understand. "Make ready, two mins."

My heart starts racing at the thought of action on the landing zone. This is something I haven't experienced yet on my tour. Watson sits across from me and pulls his helmet over his tumble of dark hair, giving me a thumbs up. I force a nervous smile.

It's a rough landing, and everyone rushes out of the chopper except me. I can't feel my legs. I feel someone grab the back of my vest and lift me up and kick me forward.

Johnny strong-arm pushes me. "Stay near the bomb dog bloke." I follow them.

I look all around for Benji, a black Lab bomb dog in the pitch black darkness. Perfect.

We run into the open field, our breathing and boots crunching in unison. My foot catches in a deep hole, tripping me. *Shit!* I catch my balance and keep running on the uneven terrain. How much mortar has this area seen? There's so much adrenaline running through me, I haven't even thought about the fact that the ground below my feet is likely littered with IEDs.

We've been told to watch where we step and never to kick anything around on the ground, but in the dark, we can't see much. Even with NVGs, this landscape is hard to navigate. We push forward as the Chinook lifts off, its engines fading to a whisper.

Just like that, the plane is gone and the reality that I am "outside the wire"—outside the safe zone where the enemy is—kicks in. The enemy could be anywhere.

I check my watch: 0200. "What's the plan then, Sergeant?" I recognize the voice coming from Vince, our sharpshooter.

Sergeant Charles answers quietly, "We'll wait here for the first morning call to prayer before we move positions."

It's oddly cold here at night, a relief from the heat of the day. "It's black as the Earl of Hell's waistcoat!" Max whispers to Mick.

"Dinnae be daft." Watson spits his tobacco into the air.

In the dark, there's continued hushed conversation for hours as I try to match names with faces. Vince is the easy one, since he has a South African accent, and Rav speaks with an intonation that sounds like music. Everyone else is Scottish, as far as I can tell.

I try to pet Benji, because he reminds me so much of Houch, but the handler stops me. "Gony, no! He works for reward, so I'm afraid you can't be pettin' him."

"Sorry." I frown and sit next to the dog, imagining I'm cuddling Houch in the comfort of my parents' house.

The murmurs settle down once the cows start to moo and animals begin stirring. I know our time to go is around the corner, and I tense up. Everything I've trained for is waiting for me now, and Sergeant Major's words stick in my mind: *Do not slow us down.*

"Prepare to move when the prayer is over," Charles says, and just then, huge speakers in the middle of nowhere blast the call to prayer for everyone in the village to hear. The very devout people in Afghanistan get up at what I consider a ridiculous hour in the morning to pray.

Once the prayer is over, that's our chance to surprise the enemy as we set out on Op Herrick, the name assigned to this mission.

For the past two months, I've heard the call to prayer multiple times a day over the loudspeaker, but this time it sounds much clearer. We must be closer to its origin.

I know we are searching for someone, but I have not been told who. I am here for a few reasons, but that reason is very much above my pay grade.

While we crouch in the grass until we can move positions, Max fills me in on previous ops. "Most of the families who have zero involvement with the Taliban leave the village when they hear fighting." He raises his lean arms into the air. "But we're bringing you along because on one of our last ops, the women stayed. The enemy began hiding phones, money, and essential materials under their burkas. Due to religious laws, the male soldiers couldn't do anything about it."

I know he's trying to make me comfortable, but it actually makes me more nervous because I have a major role to play. When he moves away to grab a cigarette, I just look at the adobe structures against the dark horizon, but then Patty starts talking.

"The structures are pure dead brilliant." He raises his thin eyebrows. "A mix of mud and straw and sticks, but so strong that a bullet from an Apache helicopter, which can go through steel, concrete, or any metal, won't penetrate it."

All around, the guys are chain-smoking and whispering, and I'm glad to release my tension when 0500 arrives and we begin pushing toward a small village not far from where we landed.

We all get into position and kick open the first door. This compound is basically sand shaped into walls. There is no furniture. There are no windows. There isn't much inside but some carpets and mats for sleeping.

I swallow hard, stand back with my weapon loaded, and observe. When Johnny kicks open the next door, screams, waving arms, and dark clothes flash before us as people flee the main room. Johnny and Rav stand square, guns drawn. Nobody's getting past them.

Unflinching, I block the path of the women and wave them into a separate room with my gun. Charles detains a few of the children, who scamper off, and forces them to my area. One mother glances behind herself at the children, and I see the panic in her eyes. I yell to the terp, "Tell the women and kids not to move and that I'll be in there soon."

The terp bawls at me and grabs me by the vest. I push him hard to the floor. "Get your hands off of me!" My face is hard, but my heart is beating fast. I've heard some terps were actually enemy combatants leading our guys into minefields, and, still shaken over the Afghan worker incident, I'm not taking any chances. It's so hard to tell the enemy from harmless civilians. Any one of these people could be armed.

As I turn toward the dusty room with the women and children, a man shouts at me in Farsi. My breathing is deep, my mind sharply focused, my gun solid and locked on him. I understand it is horrific having the military burst into your home in the early morning, so I call out to the terp, "Please tell the father I'm not going to hurt them. I just need to look around."

Suddenly an ear-splitting scream comes from the terp, waving his hands, motioning me away. In an instant, Charles is there, gun in hand, bellowing at him. I keep my eyes on everyone in the room while the muffled conversation goes on. Then Charles calls out, "Burns, take off your helmet, they think you're a man."

My hair is tucked under my helmet, and I'm wearing a scarf. I look like a small man. No wonder he's losing his mind over me going into a room with all of the women and children. The terp tells the father that I'm a woman, but he shakes his head in disbelief.

I rip off my helmet, showing off my bright blonde hair, and the man's eyes open wide. He's calmed down. The rest of my unit goes into the other rooms and searches the walls and the floors while I bring Johnny and Rav with me. "Wait outside the door while I go in with the women and kids."

It's my first time searching anyone, and I turn around, eyes taking in every detail, noticing things I've never had to pay attention to before. I'm nervous, and I'm also outnumbered by ten. I grab the oldest women first and try my best to communicate what I need them to do, which is a lot harder than it sounds.

I get all of them to spread their legs wide open, extend their arms, and face the wall.

Lives depend on me doing this right. One by one, I search the older women. I pat down their hair, and touching only the outside of their clothing, I frisk their sides, around their bras, around their feet, and inside their legs. The spots for hidden money and jewelry are endless: under their boobs, in their braids, and strapped to their legs. Having radios, excessive money was never a good sign. This almost always meant they were informing or being paid by Taliban to let them know when soldiers are in the area.

After the older women, I move on to the teenagers, some not much younger than me, who are less compliant. While I hold them against the wall, they just flop over. I don't understand what is going on. I yell out the door for a translator. "What the hell is their problem?"

He laughs.

"Hey! What are they eating?"

"A plant," he says in broken English. "They chew it and get high."

These girls are out of their trees. They have no idea what's going on, but they are still dangerous to me. They're unpredictable, and that is hazardous.

I do my best to finish searching the girls safely, but then one of them grabs at the barrel of my gun. I turn around and point it at her. "Get down!"

She plops quickly down on the dirty floor, but she's so high, she doesn't even realize what she just did.

When I'm finished with the women and girls, I turn my attention to the two children. I'm very aware of the impression I'm leaving on them. They're so little, and I don't want to scare them. They just saw me pointing a gun at their sister or cousin. Or mother? I don't know.

I smile when I approach them. I still have a job to do, but I don't have to be cruel to innocent children. With my hands off of my weapon, I put my fingers in my ears and form a funny face. This makes them smile. "I'm just going to check that you don't have anything hidden on you." I speak in a quiet, calming tone, knowing they can't understand me anyway.

Taking my fingers out of my ears but keeping the smile on my face, I start to search them, but first, I tickle them, pretending it's a game.

I hold my breath as I gently pat them down, hoping that I don't find anything on them. Thankfully, I don't. When I finish, I reach into my pocket, pull out some candy that I've been saving for an occasion like this, and press it into their warm little palms.

I take a deep breath and leave the room with the items I confiscated. "Done!" I call out to Charles while Johnny stands guard. Rav dumps the items in bags and tags them, and when we're done, Charles lowers his gun. "Braw. Let's move on."

We gather in the courtyard, and Johnny points out a cannabis plant. "They never sell these, just for personal use."

"Those girls in there were young."

"I saw a five-year-old smoking up once."

Charles lights a cigarette as he walks over to us. "We just got a call over the radio. One of the other units needs a female searcher."

Vince runs his fingers through his blaze of red hair. "We haven't seen this many women and children in the villages before."

"I know." Charles sifts through some papers. "Burns, we'll be moving you a lot more than anticipated, but the troops aren't too far apart."

All I can do is smile. I am proving to be useful to a unit, and that is all that I have ever wanted.

"We'll escort you over to the next village now." Charles tightens up his helmet. "They'll be taking over a family's compound to stay in once it gets dark so we can eat there and get some rest."

"A new area tomorrow, Sarge?" Johnny fills his gun with ammo. Charles nods.

"Pukar." Johnny points his long nose to the sky then turns to me. "The enemy likes being just close enough to watch our every movement, Burns, but not quite close enough to see us clearly."

When we reach the compound, we help to clear it. I kick in a door with my boot and come face-to-face with the barrel of a machine gun.

"Fuckin' hell!" the guy yells in a Scottish brogue. "It's the Canadian."

"Were you trying to kill me?" I scream back.

"Christ, I was guarding the door from the same enemy you're looking for!"

"You're Watson, right?"

"Aye, and you're Burns."

His sleeve is rolled up, with a bunch of tattooed letters peeking out. "What's that?"

He shows me the tattoo of his ID. "Just in case they need to identify my body."

I laugh. "What if you lose that arm?"

His blue eyes light up. "Ya rocket." And with that, he turns toward the terp. "Tell the family they have to leave so we can use their place. They'll get it back in the morning."

The family hastily gather their belongings. It's incredible how people are so willing to do what you say when you're holding a fully loaded C7 machine gun. It wouldn't have been advantageous for them to say no to us, and I believe they understood that.

One of the little girls looks up at me with terror in her dark brown eyes. She's roughly the same age as Emma, the girl from outside FOB Ramrod. I smile at her and give her a piece of candy. I never wanted to be that scary person or the soldier that scars a young child's mind.

I've heard stories from immigrants, including my own grandfather, who had soldiers storm their homes during war, and they never forgot what people did to them. While I don't want to impact an innocent person's life, war is messy, and it sounds cheesy, but that's the truth. No one wants to be the bad guy in a situation, but sometimes it's necessary. This is not a peace mission; it's a war. We can't be the nice guy.

We escort the family out, and then I wander the compound, taking it all in, especially from its high vantage point. It's my first time to inspect without any chaos. A compound has high walls with a massive square in the middle. My fingers trail the cracks on a wall that has been crumbling for years.

"Doing some cooking?" Watson's bent over a small hole two feet in the ground, his big, mischievous eyes squinting up at me. "Ya see, this is the cooking pit. The hole above it where the flames come out would be two fists either side, so a pot fits on top of it."

"How does the heat escape?"

Vince stacks wooden logs on the ground. "This little hole where the pot is. So you would leave a small other hole so the oxygen can get out and the flame doesn't go out. It's an effective way of cooking."

"Make me a cinnamon latte."

"Ya ticket!" Watson tosses a log at me, and I miss catching it, I'm laughing so hard.

"What's that?" I point to another tattoo on his arm.

"My motto. 'That others may live.'" He stands up, wiping the dirt from his pants. "I live by it every day."

As the evening wears on, I can feel myself breathing in the dust. "Johnny, how can you work out in this? I feel the sand in my teeth."

The guys roar in laughter, and Watson finally catches his breath. "He's always working out. He'll drop a push-up during firefights."

Johnny ignores us and keeps doing squats while I turn back to my meal.

"How long have you been with Black Watch?" I open my ration pack.

"A couple years." Watson takes a puff from his cigar and blows smoke out of his nostril.

"How'd you get in?"

"Family ties." He leans back on his pack. "My grandfather was a captain."

"And Sean Connery visited his granny." Vince flicks his cigarette ashes in the air.

"No way!"

"He was Grandmother's milkman." He chuckles and shakes his head. "You?"

"Nothing like that. I'm not with Canada's Black Watch regiment or anything."

Watson waves it off. "They're just styled like us." He leans back and closes his eyes. "I only joined out of rage the day after the 7/7 bombings. I'll only be doing this for four years, and then I'm going to university for journalism."

Johnny lights his cigarette and joins us. "We're Scotland's most famous military name. All the way back to the 1700s."

"Spoken like a Highland Jock." Watson tosses his shirt at him.

"Shut yer yak!" Johnny turns to me. "You're lucky to be with us, Burns."

"For the time being, so you better do more lunges. 'Cause you're getting blown up in two weeks," Watson ribs. "You're ahead of me. I'm August 10th at 1500."

"Right you are." Vince tosses his cigarette on the ground to burn itself out. "I bet ten American dollars on it."

"What?"

"Whenever there's tension, we place bets on who will get blown up and when."

"That's dark, boys!"

"Aye, but it's our best way to cope."

* * *

Gunfire breaks the stillness of the night. I jump out of my sleeping bag and race ahead with my gun. Residual smoke hangs in the air as the guys on fire watch reload.

"Now, I want you to remember that no bastard ever won a war by dying for his country." Max turns to Mick.

Mick's grin is warm, with a hint of shyness. "He won it by making the other poor dumb bastard die for his country."

Mick turns to me, and I shrug.

"*Patton*, 1970." Max lights up a cigarette to add to the smoky cloud. "Hang with us long enough, Kelsi, and you'll be able to quote every war movie ever made."

Mick flashes a toothy grin. "You can go back to sleep. The enemy retreated."

As the only female searcher they have, I'm not allowed to do any watch at night, so I don't have a fire watch shift like I did in the FOB. Fortunately for me, that means more sleep than most of the guys I'm with. It's the same deal for medics, bomb dog handlers, and the forward observers for the artillery guns.

Three hours isn't much sleep, but I've gotten by with less. I'm soaking wet with sweat and take off my kit to dry out my shirt. I grab baby wipes from my pack and have a quick "bath."

The guys are in the "pool." Some family compounds have a small river running through them or near them where we can clean up and wash laundry, but I'm more comfortable with the baby wipe method.

The rest of the unit is up early too, so we push off onto the "road" before morning prayer. I use the "road" loosely, because it is more like goat trails and tiny walkways between villages. On our way to the next village, we clear more compounds, looking for things people shouldn't have, and we find a ton of weapons, drugs, and radios.

I move carefully, in sync with my unit. Benji is ahead, and we are trusting him to guide us safely. Benji stops, we stop. Even though my legs are shorter than the guys', our pace is the same. We are one.

Scanning ahead, I watch for anything that seems out of place in this rocky and uneven terrain. Never before have I feared the ground like I do now. My throat is parched in this heat, and the thought of IEDs underfoot is more terrifying than seeing the enemy up close. At least with a human, you have a bit of an idea of what you're going up against; but with an IED, the outcome is unknown. I follow Mick and Max and am comforted by the presence of the guys behind me.

We've pushed farther and faster than we planned, and we take a break in a compound while we wait for our next orders to move.

"Your rations are weird." I chew on some pasty potato-y thing.

Mick wrinkles his freckled nose and laughs. "Not a fan of bangers and mash?"

"Does the real stuff taste like this?"

"Yeah, pretty much." Max exhales smoke into the dusty afternoon. "Except less sandy."

Spending so much time with these guys in the course of a few days has made them grow on me. When I woke to the sound of guns, I feared for them and realized how quickly someone's whole life could be taken in the blink of an eye. I hope for the best for all of us in this mud-covered compound.

A while later, Watson shakes my shoulder. "You must have been chin-strapped."

"How long did I sleep?"

"Fifteen minutes."

"The bonus of being a smaller soldier. My kit is a pillow!" I jump to my feet. "My vest pushes up, I lean my head to the side, and have a nap."

Max yells ahead. "Ready?"

We push forward along a dusty narrow road with grape fields on one side and a ditch and more fields on the other. There is a mud wall about four feet to my left and trees ahead. We set up in a compound to our right with our sniper in position, waiting for us to move forward while he provides cover.

"Tree's in the way," he radios.

Charles walks around the tree that's in the sniper's line of sight and motions over the combat engineer. "Blow it up."

He straps some explosives to the trunk, and in a few minutes, the branches fly into the air. Explosives are fun when they aren't hidden in the ground. I enjoy them when it doesn't result in any of our guys getting hurt.

It's midday at this point, and the heat is suffocating. If we move quickly, we can get to the next position and hopefully sit for a few minutes, perhaps in the shade of a tree that has not been blown up.

Just before these thoughts cross my mind, shots break through the air.

"Contact! Contact!" comes over the radio.

We are about 500 feet ahead of the position we just left, and we're getting hit from the front and flanked on the left. Mick and Max ahead of me sprint to the next wall and take cover quick.

"Push back to the position we just left," Johnny hollers above the noise. "We'll call artillery for backup."

My legs are shaking, and I feel my heart pounding. As more bullets whiz by, my whole body vibrates. Each whistle and pop, so close to my ears, scares me because I've never felt rounds this close to me.

Johnny gets in position. "Burns, you move first and I'll cover."

The enemy is close enough that I am not sticking around. "Johnny, I'm going."

"Okay, I'll count down from three—three, two, one!"

I have never run so fast in my life, and the adrenaline rush is completely exhilarating.

I have my full kit on, and I'm carrying ammo and at least six liters of water. My plates and small pack are loaded, but I am a gazelle! There is a massive hole in the ground just up ahead. It looks like an IED has gone off there at some point. There is no way around, and bullets are flying past my head, so I jump. I've grown wings and clear the hole and feel like my heart might explode. On the other side of the hole, I slide down into the ditch and wait for my next orders, my pulse loud in my ears. With one of our machine gunners providing cover, Johnny and I climb up out of the ditch and push back to the compound area. But something's wrong. The gun stops shooting. Malfunction.

I race over, crouching beneath the four-foot mud wall more easily than the other guys can. The gunner ducks down and retreats back to the compound to fix his weapon while I provide cover fire, snatching a ragged breath when I can.

We're all firing our weapons until we finally make it back to the compound. It feels like the artillery guns will never get here, but then the sound of thunder cracks through the sky, followed by a huge bang.

The big guns have got our back. Round after round flies over our heads, neutralizing the enemy. I've never experienced the role of the artillery unit from this position before, because I've always been the one shooting. The ground shakes, and I instinctively bring my hands to my ears to shield against the sound of the blast ahead. My breath catches in my throat, and I hope to God that they have the coordinates right.

"Am pure done in." Watson lights his cigar and then reaches his lighter out to Vince and Rav.

Rav curves his upper lip and starts laughing. "Wait till August 10!"

"Ya rocket." Watson turns to Charles. "Hey, Sarge, who's the sandbag tomorrow?"

"Mick."

"Give us a new movie quote, sandbag."

Pride crosses Mick face. The pride of being lead on an operation, even though it means he is the most likely to get blown up and sent home with a sandbag. "When I go home, people will ask me, 'Hey, Hoot, why do you do it, man? What, you some kinda war junkie?' You know what I'll say? I won't say a goddamn word. Why? They won't understand. They won't understand why we do it." Mick slowly turns and looks at each one of us. "They won't understand that it's about the men next to you, and that's it. That's all it is."

Smoke billows from Watson's nostril. "*Black Hawk Down*, 2001."

I look at each of these men, handsome Johnny, innocent Mick, kind Charles, pale Vince, and silly Watson. We all protected each other today. This is what it means to trust strangers, and I am very lucky to be working with such solid, reliable soldiers.

Finally, the firefight quiets down, and we all take a breather. In the stillness, Rav bursts into laughter. He's always laughing. Wish I knew what was going on in his mind.

At one point, Charles gets up, furrowing his high forehead. "We're cleared to move ahead to the next objective. Keep your eyes open for possible IEDs and signs of the enemy moving back in."

We plod along, stepping carefully, when a call comes over the radio, asking me to join another unit because they have to clear a compound filled with women. Two guys come to get me, and while I'm excited to join another unit, I'm sad to leave the guys I've bonded so strongly with.

When we enter the compound, a family greets me and begins to prepare tea. We sit down, watching the father pour water from a rusty jug into a pot.

In the meantime, we chat through the terp. Gathering intel from the people inside these small villages is vital for us to understand what the Taliban are doing and how they're controlling the areas. The better we understand the Taliban, the better we can anticipate their moves and the strategies they're using to target soldiers.

The man hands me tea in a glass cup, and I nod my thanks. But after seeing the jug that the water came out of, all I can think about is my gastro bug.

I turn to the terp. "Ask the man where his wife and children are."

"Inside," he says.

"Open the door so I can do my search." I'm wondering why he has found it necessary to lock his wife and children inside the compound.

Just then, a young girl runs out and sits with us, fixated on my blonde hair. I'm holding my camera and ask the terp, "Can this girl and I get a photo together?"

The girl beams, and we pose as I snap the camera. Afterward, I show her the image on the screen and she snatches the camera right out of my hands and runs with it into the compound, where the other women are.

"Hey!" I yell. But within a few minutes, the girl comes out holding her mother's hand, both of them smiling. As she hands the camera back to me, the terp explains, "She has never seen a photograph of herself before." I give the girl a big handful of candy.

For the first time since being here, I'm not in search mode, and I feel an actual human connection with some of these people. The sun beats down on all of us, soldier and Afghan women and children, and I can't help but smile back. This is what we're here for, to help these people lead peaceful lives.

There are the odd glimmers of hope like this, where it feels good to be seen not as a scary person here to hurt them, but rather as someone here to help.

The girl's mother points down at her ankle. She lifts her burka just a little bit to show me that she has shaved her legs. I chuckle inside. But I also realize that the Taliban could come in at any moment, and this family could switch sides, so I keep my guard up. This woman could be the very one that holds ammo under her dress, or a gun strapped to her shaved legs, who will absolutely not hesitate to kill me.

EVIL

Ohhh, you better watch yourself, Burns.

In a very short time, you'll be having nightmares about that woman and women like her.

In fact, I'll make a note to pop her into your memory now for safekeeping.

One day you'll wonder what happened to her as you think of all the "targets" you hit while you were here.

Back with the other unit, we've been moving from village to village, making good time because most of the compounds are already empty. The lack of people to search allows us to move quickly, but there must be a reason it's so quiet.

Suddenly, hot rounds zoom past us. We duck for cover and start moving to the closest compound we can find.

I run in and jump onto the roof with Vince and a few of the other guys. Lying down on our stomachs, we point our weapons to where we think the attack is coming from and shoot back.

"I'm fair puckled!" Vince runs out of ammo and lays his rifle alongside me. While he jumps down to grab another magazine, we keep firing.

With a bang, three rounds hit the weapon beside my hip, busting the buttstock wide open. Shit, that was close!

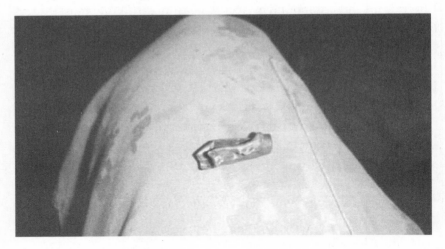

Now we're getting flanked from the left, so we reposition and return fire.

Watson cocks his head to the side, his eyes looking at the rifle then back at me. "I change my bet. You're too lucky. Ten dollars on you. September 10, a month after me!"

While Vince swears at the sight of his busted gun, the rest of us laugh as we joke around and keep firing. Deep inside, though, I know

I am one extremely fortunate soldier. The weapon just saved my hip from taking around.

I'm not even supposed to be up here, but once Noble, one of the British sergeants, told me to get up there, I knew I needed to help. As dust swirls in a trail of sun, I think back to the girl who had to shine her boots and march kilometers in the snow.

I fire another round. I'm now a soldier, and I have their backs.

June 10, 2009

"Bowfing," Mick calls out from the room, coughing and gagging.

Max laughs when he hears him moan, but upon entering the dusty room, he yelps, "Howlin!'"

Curious, I follow their voices and then cover my face with a scarf, trying not to throw up from the stench of burnt goat. Our mortar rounds hit this compound by accident last night. While mostly accurate, sometimes mortars don't land where they're supposed to. This time, a herd of goats paid the price.

"Vince," Max calls out, his trademark dimpled grin spreading across his face. "Come in out of the sun, ya fair-skinned bloke! I reckon you don't want to miss this."

Vince steps into a pile of entrails and starts swearing in a strong south African accent, "You fucking bastards," but the angrier he gets, the more difficult it is to understand him.

"You sound like an Afghan local." Mick doubles over in laughter.

Charles steps in. "We're all going to be Crabbit. We're sleeping here tonight."

"Boke!" Watson steps out of the room. "I'm away for a dauner."

I kick at the clumps of fur to see if we can clear an area, but it's everywhere. The clay floor is covered in blood and shrapnel. Mick steps over a dead goat that is mostly intact, searching a wall for contraband items. "Burns, let's have a blether, it will go faster."

I step in to join him, picking through piles of rubble that were once smooth sandstone walls. We bag and tag what we find, but it's slow going with the stench. Dear God, the smell.

"So what's your favorite war quote?"

The question takes me back home. "*Band of Brothers*."

"Pure dead brilliant."

"It was."

He looks up at me as I hold open the bag. "Oh, right." I think back to my favorite part, the line that I often kept telling myself. *I'm good at it*. "And oceans, they go up and down 'cause they have to," I start to recite, and then Mick joins me and our voices continue in unison: "I don't think we're that different. If you want to get through this, you have to start seeing it for what it is. It's something we do all the time because we're good at it.'"

GOATS

Remind Kelsi to think about what those mortar rounds do when they make contact with human beings.

Goats can be an interesting and surprising trigger.

June 11, 2009

The brim of my helmet is doing nothing to block out the heat of the sun. I'm grateful for Gould's Oakleys. I'm pretty sure I got the better deal there.

It's another day of Op Herrick, and we're moving from village to village. There's a lot of open space here, and I'm constantly scanning ahead for garbage, rock piles, anything out of place that could potentially explode.

The voices on the ICOM radio are clear, meaning the Taliban are close. We're surrounded by tall shrubbery and could be ambushed at any moment. Without a good vantage point, we somehow have to clear this area before we move the entire unit through. Right now we're in an open space, and we might as well have a target on us.

Every burka and every man is a potential threat. To say I'm on edge is the understatement of the century.

We reach an empty two-story compound on the right side of the gravel road. We send in Johnny and Watson and crouch along a mud wall on the left side. The interpreter is beside me.

"Mick, go ahead to clear the rest of this road and the hut at the end of it. It's where they go to dry grapes and roots, so there should be several women and kids there." Charles points ahead. "Then we'll move through. Max, you're his spotter. Watson and Johnny have you covered from the compound."

Charles and I hang back with two gunners until we get the okay to move. We all check our weapons, and then I start joking to break the tension. It's one thing I've learned from Watson.

"Back at KAF, I'm taking you for a real Canadian meal." I gulp some water. "Enough of the bangers and mash!"

"I'll take you for a good scoff when—"

Charles stops midsentence and holds up a hand. Our voices fall silent as sounds from the ICOM radio become crystal clear.

"The enemy is close," Charles shifts his weight. "We should—"

The earth shakes and wobbles beneath us as a muffled growl rips through the ground. I jump up to my feet as a human torso flies out of the grape hut and spins through the air.

"Fuck! Who was in there?" I scream and sit up, but Charles pulls me back.

"We can't move yet, Burns."

"Allahu Akbar," blares through the ICOM as a trail of smoke billows out of the grape hut's open roof. I don't need an interpreter to tell me what that means. They are praising God because they got one of us.

Watson's voice comes over the radio, "a string of four numbers," but I don't know whose they are. We lost a guy, but don't know who. "Hold! Hold!"

"Is that Max?" I see someone running down from the hut.

His helmet is gone, his plates are gone, his weapon is gone, his kit is gone, and he's yelling, "Where's Mick?!"

Max is bleeding from his ear, and his side is a mess.

Max's eyes dart back and forth.

"Where's Mick? Where's Mick?!" His terrified eyes meet mine. "I can't see him. Where'd he go?"

The medic bandaged Max's arms as we waited for the go to move to the grape hut. It couldn't have been his body I saw. It couldn't.

As they carry Max into the compound, his voice still rings out, "Where's Mick?"

Suddenly, the firing starts. The Taliban's been watching from the tree line, and now they're shooting at us. We're taking mortar rounds—heavy fire. I jump into the ditch with Charles and two machine gunners.

"We can't take the road, but we've got to get Mick," Charles cries through quick breaths. He motions to the gunners. "Cover us at the door of the hut."

My breath, my heart, everything slams loud in my ear, but the world is silent to me, despite the gunfire. I feel like I'm underwater.

The gunners run ahead and start shooting to provide cover for us. Charles touches my arm. "On three: one, two, three!"

We run as fast as we can, directly into the grape hut. It's shady in here, but light comes in through the cracks in the wall and the giant hole in the ceiling. The walls and ceiling are made from mud and sticks, with rectangular holes in the walls allowing for circulation. It's like I'm stuck inside a giant wooden cheese grater, and that's when I see shredded chunks of human flesh clinging to the walls of the hut.

Pieces of kit and body dangle from the ceiling and cover the floor. There's a smell in the air, the char of burnt flesh. I wobble, and my head feels tight, as if something's squeezing down on it. I stare at a piece of skin draped from a stick, look right through it, and a surge goes through my head, releasing my brain into a void. I feel nothing.

Charles puts his hand on my shoulder. "Are you all right, Burns?"

"Where's Mick?" I ask, looking around.

"Whatever's here, is here," mumbles Charles.

I see the hole at the back of the hut where the IED went off and reach inside. "Where is he?"

I pull out a boot, still fully laced with a foot and calf in it. "Well, at least the boot is still good." I turn to Charles.

"I'll take that." Charles snatches the boot from me.

I will never be proud of that moment, but something in my brain broke—those words came out as a coping mechanism, not out of disrespect. My light switch turned off in the moment.

No man or woman gets left behind, so we gather pieces of Mick in plastic evidence bags. I have no gloves and use my bare hands to pull pieces of flesh, bone, and other pieces out of the walls and into the bags. I grab his helmet and try not to look at what I pour out of it.

"Contact!" Mortar rounds fly down and bullets whiz by, shaking the grape hut walls. Charles calls for support as we put what we collected of Mick on a stretcher. The enemy is using this opportunity to attack, and we're taking heavy fire. I pick up pieces of flesh and mindlessly stuff them in my pockets. I strap Mick's helmet and rifle onto myself, along with Max's whole kit since it was blown off in the blast, onto the stretcher. Everything is covered in dirt and blood. Charles and I run to the angel flight coming to collect the dead and injured.

They're shooting heavy, and our Black Hawk circles around just in time, unleashing rounds out of the doors. *Ratttttattttattttt*, and they clear out the Taliban.

We run as fast as we can, carrying one stretcher containing parts of Mick. One of the gunners carrying Mick trips and drops his end of the stretcher, and parts of the man fall to the ground. We pile everything back on, trying to hide what's happening from Max. We're running, and shots are whizzing past us. We're out in the open, and I have no idea how the shots are missing us as hot brass rains down and peppers the ground. Whistle, pop. Whistle, pop.

We put a tarp over Mick's stretcher and position Max right beside it.

"Where's Mick?" Max keeps asking.

"Don't worry!" we reassure him. "We have him."

"Where's Mick?"

"Don't stress. We've got him."

The angel flight takes off, and once the door gunners make their presence known again, the firefight dies down.

Back in the compound, everyone is chain-smoking, puffing into the quiet air. The firefight is over. They got our brother, and they deserved what they got from the Black Hawk.

I hold out my hand. "I need a cigarette."

"You don't smoke, Burns." Watson bites down on his cigar. "We're not gonna let you start now."

My hands are covered in blood. I wipe them on my legs and my chest but can't remove it. "I can't get it off. I can't get it off!"

CONTACT

I've got her.

The pretty little blonde one.

I took a couple of the other guys too, but they won't *admit it*.

And you know what will happen, then?

They'll do the heavy lifting for me, if you catch my drift.

This one is feisty, and she'll put up a good *fight*.

Did you see the look on her face when I entered her brain?

Ha ha ha ha.

She isn't even twenty years old, and she's *mine* now.

Forever.

Let's see.

Kelsi.

How shall I fuck with you…

You'll obviously *never* touch Jell-O or raw meat again.

And I made your brain process the *smell* of him
as a piece of fresh pork.

Bye-bye, Grandma's Hungarian ham.

It's the details, you see.

That's how I maintain *control*.

Rub your hands with as much hand sanitizer as you
like now.

You'll never stomach the smell of it again.

Now that I'm in, I have *access* to your brain's wiring.

And now I *play*.

I stare down at my kit and my hands covered in dirt and blood. Blood from Mick and Max. I wipe my hands rapidly over my vest and pants, pour water over them, and rub as hard as I can.

All I can think about is the color and the smell of the blood, and I can't get it off.

The way Mick's flesh felt like a piece of raw meat in my hand. I can't stop thinking about it.

IMPRINT

Did you feel it, Kelsi?

I've imprinted all of this in your mind's eye.

Like a movie you can never turn off.

A picture on the back of your eyelids.

You won't stop thinking about this day.

It's impossible.

Every single time you close your eyes, I'll turn
on the memory reel.

You make the popcorn. Just don't *burn* it.

Within twenty minutes of the Black Hawks taking off and heading back to KAF, we organize and move out. To get to our next objective, we have to walk along the same road, past the same grape hut we just picked Mick out of.

HANDS

What's that on your hands, Kelsi?

You should go wash up.

Make sure to get all the blood out from under your fingernails.

My hands are all I focus on as we tread carefully along the road. I follow Charles and Watson and keep rubbing my fingers to get the blood off. These guys have all seen things like this before, and it's business as usual for them, so I try to play it cool. While they joke around, I have to be tough and push forward.

We walk by the grape hut, slowly, with our eyes wide open. I hold my breath the entire time, reliving the fearful blow of the explosion, seeing Mick's body splayed throughout the building, hearing Max's panicked cry.

Finally, we make it through the area and onto the road that will take us to the next village. I'm hoping I can put all this behind me. Some part of me knows that I won't, but I try anyway.

June 12, 2009

For the next day, we walk and walk, until the familiar whistle crack of gunfire sounds.

Again.

We duck into a compound that's thankfully empty. Charles organizes the fire watch and sends me to a room to rest. I don't have the energy to argue. We take more rounds throughout the night, but nothing the machine gunners and air support can't handle.

Bullets whizzing through the air has become a calming noise that rocks me to sleep, like a lullaby. Those sounds are a comfort, because I can tell how far away the enemy is and whether or not I need to run and take cover, or if they are just loud echoes of rounds from afar.

It's not like I can sleep anyway. Whenever I close my eyes, the nightmares come.

SWEET DREAMS

```
Trouble sleeping, Kelsi?

But why?

Are you thinking about Mick?

Or, how if it weren't for Vince's weapon, you might
be dead or paralyzed?

Or about the Taliban hiding outside the walls,
waiting to blow you up?

Ready to go home yet, Burns?
```

June 13, 2009

The next day, we move to a smaller village, where we clear a few compounds and find more ammunition, weapons, and drugs.

We confiscate anything that can possibly be traded to the Taliban. They can't ambush us if they don't have the money or weapons to do so, and we don't want them to have any more means to be able to kill us.

The deeper we get, the more we find, and our days and nights are so busy that there isn't time to think. I like it that way.

I haven't thought for days about how bad I smell, and I'm getting comfortable with how disgusting I am. Tonight, for example, I'm ready to nap with cows and chickens.

Under the cover of night we move into the field beside the compound we've occupied, waiting for a Chinook to drop a shipment of water and food for our unit.

With our NVGs, we lie on our stomachs, in the prone position, watching for the flashing light on the bottom of the helicopter.

Finally, the whisper of blades sounds in the distance, and we see it coming over the mountain. Once overhead, the chopper drops extra ammo, rations, and enough water to last us a few days. They're in and out quick so they don't give our position away to the enemy.

June 14, 2009

I bring my boot up high and kick the door in. The same scene again and again. Screaming and shouting; people running around scared. We've been at this nonstop for the last few days without much rest. We gather up the women and children to be searched, and I direct them all in one room, with the help of a terp.

I go through my usual routine, putting the older women against the wall first, but this time something feels off. Each group is different at each compound, but the women and kids in this particular home are a lot angrier than those I've encountered before. These women have a wild look in their eyes, and they aren't very cooperative.

The hair on the back of my neck stands up as my body senses danger. Before I start my search, I turn to the guys. "Something's not right. Please stay close to the door and listen for me, with a terp."

Watson steps in front of the door. "You got it, Burns."

"Thanks." I turn to Johnny, who is holding the metal detector. "Can you clear an area so I can pee?"

He walks ahead and sweeps the metal detector back and forth, but loud beeps come through. "Okay, not here."

Then again two feet to the right, more beeps.

"Okay, go right there." He points to a small spot. "And don't move to either side if you want to keep your legs. I'll turn my head."

I don't question him. I turn around, pee, and quickly move back to the part of the compound where the women are waiting.

As I open the door, I hear a loud bang.

"What the hell was that?"

Watson is right behind me as a mother repeatedly kicks at the door and then spits on me.

"That's a bad fucking idea!" I grab her arms, throw her to the ground, put her arms behind her back, and zip-tie her wrists. She struggles. "Sit still!"

She can't understand me whatsoever and continues to kick, scream, and spit. The teenagers in the room start pacing, and I am outnumbered. I poke my head out the door and call out, "Can I get some help in here?"

The terp laughs and walks away, but I call after him, "Hey, you piece of shit. Stand by the door and do your job."

He doesn't like being spoken to by a woman this way and just folds his arms and looks away. I get no respect, but my Brits have my back.

I turn back to the women, one glaring at me wild-eyed through the screen in her burka. To my right I hear heavy footsteps, and a woman runs at me with giant metal shears. I look her square in the eyes and raise my weapon. She doesn't stop, so I hit her in the face with the butt stock of my gun, and she drops like a bag of potatoes. It's the best outcome for her in this moment; I could have shot her.

I grab her, tie her arms behind her back, and sit her down. "Stay right here, or you're going to get bagged." I turn to the terp. "Translate that."

I push through the room, banging my hands along the walls and under the sheets that hang in the home. From several hidden compartments, I pull out money, the Qur'an, gold, jewelry, and a bunch of cell phones. Despite protocol that dictates I should place all items in full view of the detainees, I throw a few things out the door. Since one of them just tried to stab me in the face, I'm not in the mood to respect their property.

Thankfully, this is the last search. We head to the next empty compound, eat, clean our weapons, and wait for our orders. It's time to go back to KAF for our debriefing.

As the last hours of the op are closing in, I sit with my guys. Nobody says much. Rav doesn't break out in his habitual laughter, and Johnny isn't even exercising. Vince stares at the wall, and Charles cleans his gun. Watson doesn't crack one joke and just writes in his war journal as he puffs on a cigar. All are chain-smoking, and I just sit and stare at the wall.

The call comes through, and Charles gets up. "Let's move to the LZ [landing zone], but proceed with caution. We're sitting ducks in the middle of an open field in the Panjwai district."

"What else is new?" Watson tosses his cigar on the ground.

Rav lifts the heavy bags. "We've got Chinooks?"

Charles nods. "Two."

In the distance, we hear our lift, the Chinooks are coming.

SCISSORS

That was close. I'll add this one to your memory reel.

Every time you cut something—the string to a bag of onions or the ribbon to a wrapped gift.

Every time someone hands you scissors, I'll be there.

For hours we're "safe" in the air, but everyone is totally silent. I can't close my eyes, because like a VHS tape rewinding and replaying, I see everything over and over. No matter how much I desperately try to shake the image of Mick's body flying through the air, I can't. It's a hologram in front of my eyes—virtual reality that I can't control or turn off.

FLASHBACK

    Play it again.
    Again.
    Again.

It's late when we land inside KAF. We all unload onto the safety of the tarmac. I have never been so happy to be on solid ground—or at least on a field that has no explosives underneath it. I'm told by the British MPs that I can go, but I have to report to their offices in the morning for a debrief since I've been involved in several events during the operation.

There are supposed to be some Canadians from my unit waiting to take me the five or six kilometers back to the Canadian side of KAF, but there's nobody here besides me. I walk to my barracks, alone, accompanied by the image of Mick. No matter how I try to distract myself with thoughts of home, my friends, the beach—I see his torso flying through the air, and I'm back inside the grape hut.

I'm exhausted, my clothes are stained with someone else's blood, and the only thought I can latch onto that distracts me is the thought of going back out to get my revenge.

WISHFUL THINKING

You aren't going to get that image out of your head.

Not today.

Not tonight.

Not tomorrow.

Not ever.

Doesn't work that way, kiddo.

I have you now, and I won't let go.

Those things you just saw/heard/smelled/felt?

They're with you forever.

That's how I make sure you and I never part.

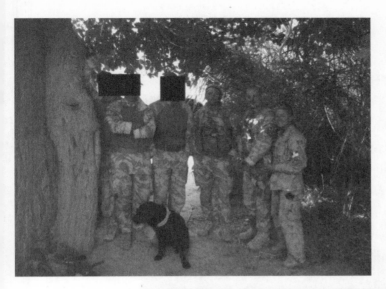

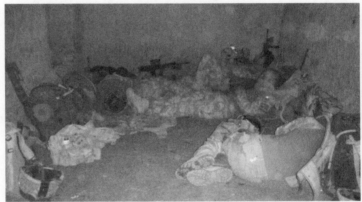

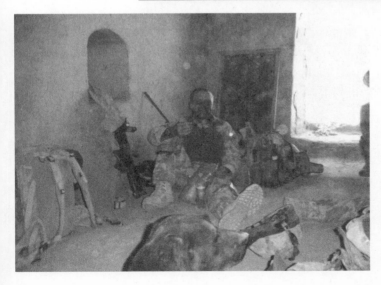

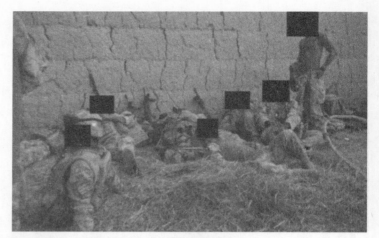

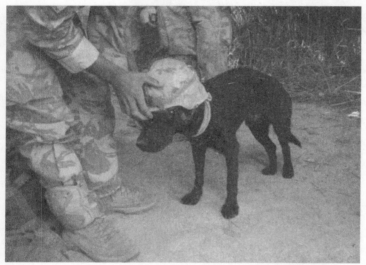

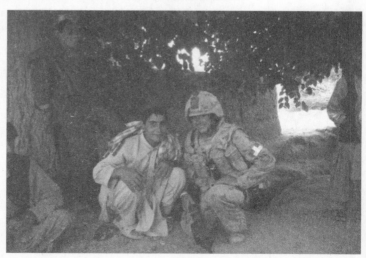

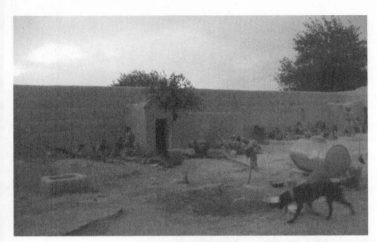

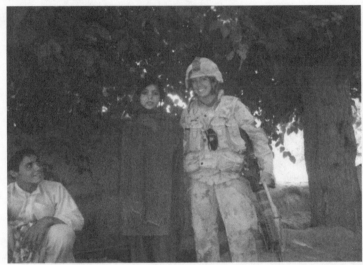

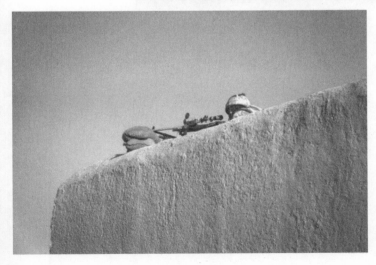

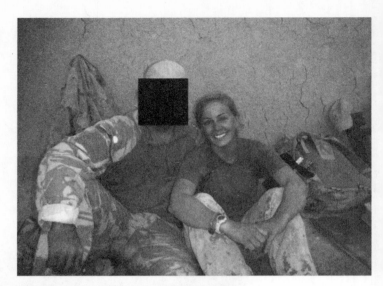

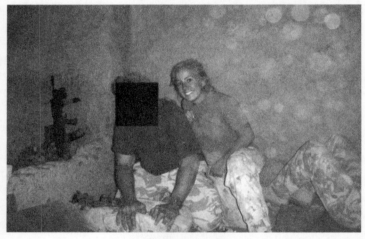

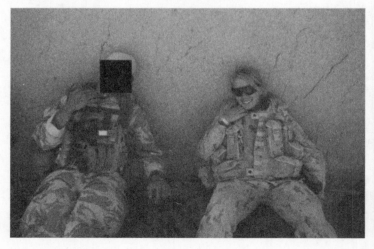

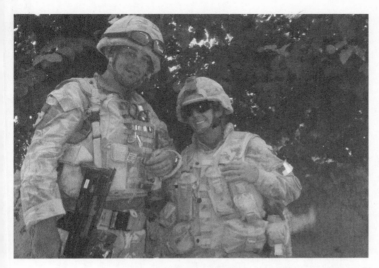

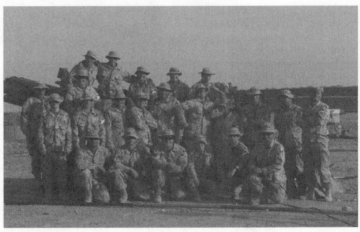

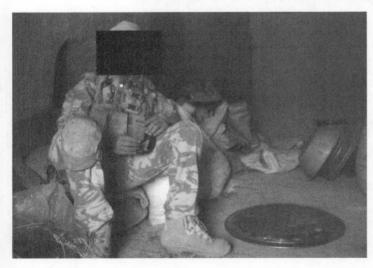

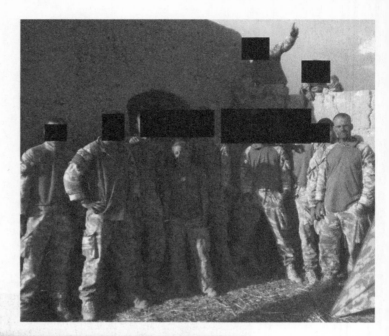

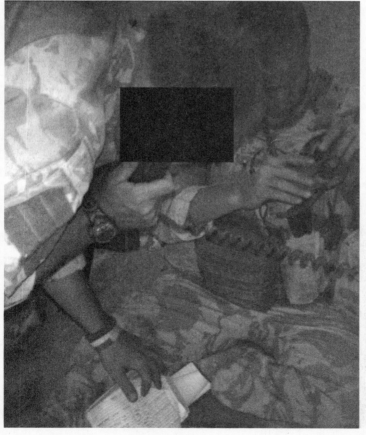

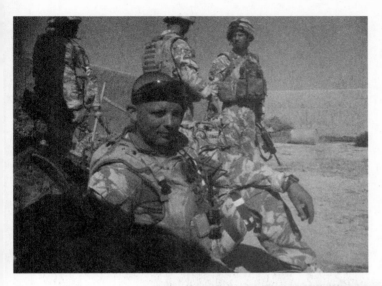

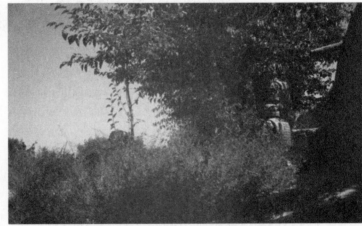

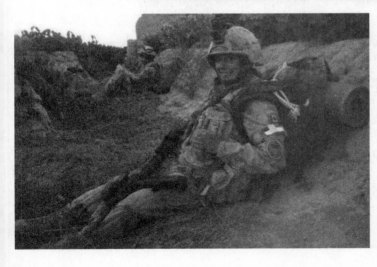

TWELVE

Post Op

The moment I close the door, tears sting my eyes and soak my face. A week's worth of emotion pours out of me, and my chest heaves.

The sour stench of sweat and the metallic smell of blood fill the safety of my room at KAF. I've been in the same clothes for a week, and I can't get them off fast enough.

For four days, I've slept, eaten, and breathed in this bloodstained kit. Parts of Mick have been in these pockets. I can still feel his warm flesh in my hands.

In the bathroom, I lock the door and stare at myself in the mirror. *Who are you, with the sunburnt cheeks, smeared with tears and dirt? Are you really still only nineteen? Those eyes have seen too much.*

I pull the elastic from my hair and take out the three-day old braid. Sand falls all over the floor. God, I hate sand.

My boots are a mess. I haven't actually looked at them in a while. They have holes on both sides, and the duct tape holding them together is fraying. I shake the boots out; rocks and dirt spill onto the floor. I hate rocks.

Stripping down to bare skin, I turn on the shower—as hot as it will go.

My head spins the second I stand under the water, and I slide down the wall onto the shower floor. Water is rationed here, but I only let myself worry about that for a second because I can't move.

I need the sound of mortars to calm me down, but all I can hear is Max screaming for Mick. My body shakes with fear as the terror replays in my head. I close my eyes, but I can still see Mick's sweet, smiling face. No matter how much I wash, I can't get the blood off my hands. My chest heaves with raging sobs until I can't catch my breath, and I cry until I feel an emptiness as raw as the skin I'm scrubbing.

GOOD GIRL

You're a fast learner, Kelsi.

You already know how this is going to work.

Every

Time

You

Close

Your

Eyes

You

See

It.

You smell it.

You taste it.

You feel it.

Know how to make it stop?

Lights out.

Water pours down over me, and the shower floor is covered in sand, filth, and remnants of blood. I tuck my knees to my chest and cry in the fetal position, staying there until the water runs cold.

My skin is covered in goose bumps, and I reach up and turn off the tap. Still dizzy, I catch my balance as I step out of the shower and lean against the wall. Shivering, I grab a towel and scream at the top of my lungs.

I thought I was out of tears.

SERVICE BULLETIN

> Nobody's coming to comfort you.
>
> No Mommy or Daddy.
>
> No Dillon.
>
> No Jen or Bine.
>
> No Mick.

Somehow, I manage to reach the bed, but I don't have the energy to get dressed. I pull the damp towel around myself, bring the covers up to my head, tuck my knees into my chest, and sob.

I wish my parents were here.

I wish I was home so that Dad could tell me everything's going to be okay and Mom could hug me through it.

I can't close my eyes, because that's where the nightmares hide.

June 15, 2009

For three days I wake up at 0430 and go to my debrief with the British MPs. I'm told it's routine to make sure everyone's stories line up and everything is clear, but I'm wearing thin.

I wear the same disgusting, filthy boots, stained with blood. They must smell it during questioning.

"Where was Mick's body found?"

"The grape hut."

"Who was with Mick when he died?"

"Max was the only one in the grape hut, that I could see."

"How many people were with you when Mick died?"

I count on my fingers. "Charles, Watson, Max—" I stop for a moment and look at the clock. This will probably be another six-hour interrogation. How many rounds were fired? Who was there? In what order did events occur? How did we run into the firefight? This British MP is thorough, but over and over again? Each day she writes down my statement, wanting to know all the details about the op, every incident. Every little detail.

"Where was each piece of his body found?"

"The grape hut. In the ceiling, the walls, the hole where the IED went off."

Why do they keep making me go through this? Don't they know they are adding scenes to the horror movie that will play in my head for the rest of my life? Why are they making me relive and repeat a moment I will never forget, but desperately want to?

For the rest of the day I'm on autopilot, trying my best to recall what time things happened, who was there, how many rounds were fired, who handled what, when we started getting contact.

Until it's time for Mick's ramp ceremony.

Two hundred soldiers parade onto the tarmac, each looking resolutely in front of them, lost in their own world, without noticing the emotion of others around them.

My unit is brought right up in front, and a lump rises in my throat when I see the Brits. Tears run down Watson's face, and our eyes meet. Charles, Rav, and Vince all let their eyes well up as if proud to shed a tear for Mick, who had their back. Even cocky Johnny doesn't hide his wet face, as if those tears are his salute to Mick, to his family back home.

I stand alone in my marching row—behind the Brits and in front of the Canadians—waiting for the command to go to attention as the caskets get closer to the Herc. Besides Mick, there's a thirty-five-year-old Canadian, Corporal Joseph Robert Martin Dube.

It's time to say our last goodbyes to the people we lost on our op and send them home to their families.

The haunting sound of a lone bagpipe playing "Flowers o' the Forest" moves closer, and on one long, continuous note, six soldiers carrying the casket stop. They place one hand each on the back of their comrade, linking them as one.

I step into position and stand at attention. When the call comes for the final salute and 200 soldiers in the hangar lift their arms in unison to salute our friend, my legs buckle. I can't support my own weight, and two women grab me from behind to hold me.

My eyes drift to Mick's casket, and I know how little of him is inside.

Tears fall heavy and fast as I try to call out, but my voice balls up in my throat. For a moment, my legs grow heavy, pushing my voice through until I feel as if I can't stand. "He isn't even in there," I say to myself. Salt from my tears sting my chapped lips, and as much as I try, I can't catch my breath.

The bagpipe plays over my sobs as the casket is draped in the British flag and loaded into the Herc. There's a weight on my chest, and it's crushing my lungs and heart.

The soldiers lower their salute. Some go to say goodbye, telling Mick, "See you in Valhalla, brother," and "See you in the re-org." I want to join them, but I'm still on my knees, wailing, hands pressed into the grit, leaning against someone's leg. The two women are trying to hold me up and help me calm down. Their voices are soothing, but I know Mick's casket is filled with sandbags to mimic the weight of his body, and I am sick.

SANDBAGS

> Heads up, Kelsi.
>
> That ramp ceremony?
>
> It's going to fuck you up for the rest of your life.
>
> You'll never hear a bagpipe again without thinking of Mick's parents burying a casket full of sand.
>
> Oh, and by the way, you won't see anyone in Valhalla.
>
> That's where the warriors go in the afterlife.
>
> And you're a weak little girl.

Two days after the ceremony, after my three days of questioning are over, I am invited to the Brits' barbecue. The smell of meat searing on the grill turns my stomach, and I force down the bile.

Charles walks over to me first, a vacant look on his face. "Thanks for coming, Burns."

"A somber party." Watson hands me a beer. "But Mick would have wanted us to keep our barbecue."

"Mick had gumption, barreling into that grape hut with the metal detector. He'd be so proud knowing he saved the rest of us."

Johnny lets out a deep sigh, his T-shirt pulled tight against his chest. Everyone is in civilian clothes, and I feel out of place in my uniform. I figured because the barbecue was on base, I needed to be in uniform. No one told me this was informal.

Watson lights up his cigar. "He had our back."

Vince nods and starts to recite, "When I go home people will ask me, 'Hey Hoot, why do you do it, man? What, you some kinda war junkie?'" He looks to Johnny.

Johnny takes a long puff and watches the smoke curl. "You know what I'll say? I won't say a goddamn word. Why?" He looks to Rav. Rav presses the cigarette to his lips and takes a deep drag. "They won't understand. They won't understand why we do it." He turns to Charles.

"They won't understand that it's about the men next to you, and that's it." Charles pauses. "That's all it is."

I've been quiet all along, but I find the strength to say four words. "*Black Hawk Down*, 2001."

We all stand in silence, looking down at our feet, then up toward the flag blowing in the wind.

"Aye, Mick." Watson tilts his bottle. "See you in the re-org!" Charles raises his beer. "Yeah, Vikings."

I lift mine, and we all join in and drink to our friend.

We stand quietly again, each of us with a distant stare, united in that one moment none of us can shake. Even when we eat, chomping and slurping just fills the void. I nibble at my food while the guys gulp theirs down. Once in a while, a sliver of conversation breaks through.

"They're done questioning you?"

"Yep."

"The British cleared everyone involved." Charles swigs a beer. "Made sure we all had the same story."

There's a lull again until Johnny puts down a lobster tail. "It's disgusting."

Vince nods and does the same. "Hot on the outside and frozen on the inside."

"The steak was better." Watson spits his tobacco. "One of us will probably die from it."

"Not you." Johnny holds out his cigarette. "It's not August yet."

The guys crack up, and I just pour the beer down my throat. In our line of work, we have the darkest humor, but I can't force words out of my mouth or find a smile to cross my face. I haven't slept. Maybe that's it.

We all fall quiet again until Rav asks, "How's Max?" Not long ago, his beautiful sing-song voice made me smile, but now I just stare blank-faced. *Mick should be here*, is all I keep thinking.

"Not sure." Charles flicks ashes onto the ground. "He was flown back to the UK to have his lacerations looked after."

I find my voice. "He won't lose his arm, will he?"

"Nah."

"A friend of mine got both his legs blown off on tour." Watson sends a puff of smoke through his flaring nostril. "I was the medic that dealt with him. He said to me, 'Do you mind if I borrow your trainers?'" Everyone starts laughing, and he holds his cigar in the air. "I go back to base. Sent him *Runners Weekly*, socks, and shoes." He's buckling over in laughter with the guys. "Bit the legs off of gummy bears and sent them to him."

I know they use dark humor to stay one step darker than the actual situation they're facing. This keeps them sane, but all I keep thinking of is Mick. I can't laugh. I can't think of anything other than him. He was just a kid. The same age as me. I could have easily been the one to step on that IED. Why wasn't it me?

I realize they're all looking at me as if I'm made of glass. Like I could break at any moment.

GLASS

    Silly girl.
    You're already broken.
    And beyond repair.

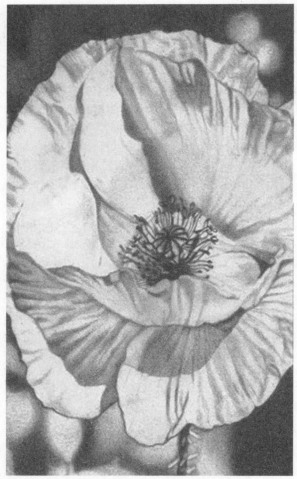

Poppy, Vanessa Sheren. Drawn by my sister-in-law.
This is tattooed on me.

PART 2

UNITY

THIRTEEN

All the Meds

"I can't do this anymore." I look the military doctor square in the eye. "I can't sleep. I can't stop crying. I lay in bed at night just waiting for the sun to come up."

He scribbles notes in my file and leans back in his chair. "Kelsi, you have acute post-traumatic stress disorder. It's going to take some time."

"How much time? I've been here for two weeks. I'm yelling and swearing at everyone, including the officers, and that's going to get me in big trouble. I need to get out of KAF and back on the guns at Ramrod."

"We'll get you back there in time, but first you need to take your HLTA. Where are you going for your decompression?" Home Leave Travel Assistance was something the Army did to give us decompression time as needed so we got to go on a break wherever we wanted for two to three weeks during our tour.

"The Dominican with my mom for three weeks, but I can't go like this. I'm in no shape to see anyone," I admitted.

"You have to go. We'll adjust your medication so you can start sleeping, and then you'll feel better."

"But what's the point? I don't want to leave. My mom will just be worried seeing me like this."

He shoves a bottle of pills across the desk. "They're very fast-acting, so go right to bed when you take them."

The thought of sleep is terrifying. It means closing my eyes, and when I do that, the same horror movie plays over and over and over again.

MEDICATE

```
That's it, Kelsi.
Take the pills.
Numb your brain.
The weaker you are, the more power I gain.
```

I know that the medication worked because I have no memory of getting myself from Dubai to Paris to Toronto and then to the Dominican Republic. The driver drops me off at the resort. "Enjoy your holiday, Miss. It's nice and hot here in July."

Slamming the door without saying anything, I lug my bag to the entrance. I scan my surroundings, trying to spot my mother, but there's no sign of her. It's beautiful here, with vibrant flowers and tall palm trees, but I can't force a smile.

Adjusting Gould's Oakleys, I take a deep breath and walk into the resort, wondering how Gould and McMillin are doing. And Bless. And all my Brits.

Inside the lobby, Mom is sitting on the edge of a wicker chair with her eyes fixed on the door. When she sees me, she jumps up and runs over. "Kelsi! How were your flights?" She pulls me into a huge hug. "Oh, my little girl. It's so good to have you back in one piece."

I can't manage to hug her back. She has no idea how many pieces her daughter is in right now and that there's not enough glue in the world to hold them all together.

My body goes limp after a minute, prompting her to pull away. "Are you okay, hon?"

No matter how hard I try to pull my lips up at the corners, I can't do it. I can't smile. Nor can I find any words to answer her. The best I can do is stare straight ahead with my eyebrows pulled together so tightly that I have a headache.

"Let's go to our room and get you settled," she says. "I think you could use a drink."

Pull it together for her, Kels.

Walking through the resort, I sense that someone's watching me. Pulling my sunglasses over my hair like a headband, I check over my left shoulder, my right shoulder, then left again as Mom chats with the front desk person. Edging along the wall, I turn a corner fast, my fingers tracing the switchblade in my pocket. All I see is a lobby full of tourists. How can they look so happy when there's so much shit going on in the real world? Do they even know what's happening in Afghanistan? Do they have any idea of how many people are dying today to fight for their freedom?

I skulk toward the window and take a wide step around a crumpled newspaper on the floor. My eyes scan for more IEDs, on the floor, on the beach. *There are no bombs here, Kelsi. You're not there anymore. And God, how did you get through security with a knife?* Outside, women walk around in bikinis, and the only thing men hold are cold drinks. For a moment, I watch a child building a sandcastle under the protection of a sunburst umbrella. *I hate sand.* Then a gecko scurries up the wall, and I'm back in Afghanistan.

Closing my eyes, I am in the desert, sweating under the weight of my kit and my weapons. I miss it and hate it all at once.

FLASHBACK

Look, Kelsi, a turban!

That bastard might have a gun…or a knife!

He wants to kill you.

You better protect yourself.

But you're unarmed, aren't you?

Go have a Rum & Coke.

My eyes dart back and forth, and I rush to the reception desk, wringing my hands and pacing. There's a pitcher of ice water on the counter, and I pour myself a glass, drink it, and breathe. Mom glances over at me with a furrowed brow and waves goodbye to the front desk attendant. Her smile falls when she looks at me. "Let's go, honey. You must be tired."

No matter how tired I am, I no longer sleep. If only I could tell her that, but my brain can't find the words.

EXHAUSTION

Tsk, tsk, Kelsi.

Disappointing your mother.

Look at the pain in her eyes.

It's so hard for her to pretend she loves you as she used to.

Before your "incident" in Afghanistan.

Want to hear a secret?

She's already mourning you.

Why are you trying so hard to keep going?

At dinner, despite a nap, nothing has changed. I look around nervously and pull back whenever a waiter approaches our table.

"Aren't you hungry?" Mom holds her knife and fork above her place setting.

A server drops a metal dish, and I jump as the clang echoes through the dining room. Sitting back farther in my chair, staring at my plate, I drag a French fry through a blob of ketchup and put in my mouth. "Not really."

A fleeting sigh passes through Mom's lips before she starts talking. "The fish is really good. Want to try some?"

She pulls her fork back when I shake my head, and she slowly chews. We sit in silence for a while, me shoving fries around on my plate, her slicing through her fish and potatoes. I keep watching a family sitting at a nearby table, laughing and smiling. They look so happy, and I wish I could be like that again. Will I ever?

My beer is almost empty, and I take a long drink.

"How about we head back to our room if you're not hungry, Kels? Maybe we can watch a movie?"

"Sure, Mom. Whatever you want." I bring the beer to my lips and pour the cold bitterness down my throat. "Just let me finish this." One more swig, and I place the bottle next to another empty one.

As we walk to our room, I focus on the stars instead of the sand beneath my feet. The feel of each kernel between my toes or in my hair takes me right back to Afghanistan. Sadly, even the night sky will never be beautiful to me again. Everything is tainted by thoughts of Mick. Hopefully the beer buzz helps me sleep tonight.

"You're sure you don't want to talk about it?" Mom asks.

I shake my head and stumble. Mom reaches out to catch me. "Oops. Your alcohol tolerance must be pretty low. Be careful!"

Back in the room, Mom fixes some tea while I start unpacking my bag, folding my clothes and putting them away. She chats with me from the other room. "I'm doing a bit more trucking on my own these days, did I mention that?"

My hands move slowly, thanks to the alcohol, as I lay my socks together. I fold them in half, fold them again, and tuck the ends in. "That's nice." I struggle to think of something else to say. "Good for Dad to have a break now and then."

"Now that you and Dillon don't need me around as much, it makes sense for both of us to be working. Plenty of bills to be paid."

I put the socks in neat rows in my top drawer and count them. "Uh-huh."

For a minute, Mom doesn't say anything. She's watching me from the doorway.

"What?" I ask sharply.

"Nothing."

She goes into the living room, turning on the light.

"What are you *doing*?" I run over to the switch, yelling, "Turn it off! You can't have lights on right now!"

"Kelsi, what are you talking about?" Her hands rise to her face. We stand in the dark.

Shit, I've frightened her. I'm being irrational. "Never mind, Mom," I switch on the light then give her a hug. "Sorry. It's just a rule we had over there. I'm sorry. I'm not myself right now."

She clings to me until my BlackBerry buzzes and I pull away. It's Brady:

Can't stop thinking about you.

I write back:

Pls don't stop.

It's so easy to talk to him. He never asks any questions about what I've been doing on my tour, which makes it easy to forget. I feel like I could open up to him if I wanted to. But Mom? If she knew about the things I've done, she would never love me again.

The bathroom door closes, and I hear Mom crying above the sound of the exhaust fan.

Brady messages right back:

I couldn't even if I tried. I want to see you when you get back to Canada.

i can't wait. but i'm warning you, i'm a mess.
lol i need to get some sleep. xo

Sweet dreams, babe.

i wish.

Grabbing a beer from the mini bar, I crack it open and use it to chase down my sleeping meds before curling into a ball on the bed and crying into my pillow. When I sleep, the nightmares will come. I wish I could crawl in bed with Mom like I did when we traveled for Tae Kwon Do tournaments. She always calmed my nerves, but nothing can now. She's such a good mom and deserves a better daughter than I now can be. At least she has Dillon, one normal child.

At breakfast, I order a second mimosa to go with my bacon and eggs.

"What should we do today, kiddo?"

"Whatever you want," I say, my eyes glued to the TV screen showing news from Afghanistan.

Mom takes a drink of coffee. "Dillon's excited to see you again." A text from Brady momentarily takes my attention away from the TV:

Dreamt about you. You were naughty.

I smile and start to tap a response.

"Who's that?" Mom asks.

"Just Brady."

"Brady?"

"The guy I met in Montreal."

"Oh, I didn't think that was serious."

"It's not."

"Okay." She picks up a newspaper and pretends to read it, but I can see her watching me. I know I'm the reason her forehead is wrinkled into a frown.

At the end of three weeks, I've been drunk a handful of times, followed the news to see who's been dying in Afghanistan (three from our unit), shed a million tears, fantasized about my death, and tried to smile for my mother. She's heard me crying and doesn't know what to do with me, but I can't help her. It's hard enough to keep myself standing upright, and I'm grateful she respects me enough not to push the conversation. I can't wait to get myself on the first flight back to Dubai. Ramrod is home now.

YOUR FAULT

You can safely assume from now on, that any time your parents are upset, it's because of you.

You messed up the family.

Your role was supposed to be "darling daughter," but what's this you're giving them?

Know how you've been fantasizing about death all the time?

Do everyone a favor.

Give them a real reason to grieve.

FOURTEEN

Cracked

Holding the wall for balance, I pull my right ankle toward my tailbone for a deep quad stretch while Sergeant Leblond puts our dumbbells away.

"How are you doing, Burns?"

I release my right foot and shift my weight to stretch the other leg. "Fine. My hips seem a bit tight."

"I don't mean physically."

"Well what *do* you mean?" I snap, dropping my foot.

"Kelsi…" He walks away from the dumbbells and sits down on the bench, waiting for me to answer.

"What? What do you want me to say?"

"You were involved in an op that killed one of your guys, and you watched it happen." His voice is gentle. "How are you doing with that?"

"I appreciate your concern and all, Sergeant, but I saw shit and I have to deal with it. I don't know what to tell you."

"If you need anything, come talk to me?"

I clench my jaw. "If we're done here, I have to go meet Gould."

Plodding down the dusty path, I consider going back to apologize to Sergeant Leblond when Gould calls out from the top of the laundry tent. "Hey! Forgot about me?"

"Sorry, I'm in my own world these days." I drop my bag on the floor.

"That's understandable. You've been through some heavy shit. I know what it's like out there."

I nod without saying anything. Gould has done a few tours with McMillin. He saw his buddies die—he told me about it. Maybe I should talk to him about McMillin, but I just can't. At least not yet. Gould's voice breaks the awkward silence. "So what were the Brits like?"

"Solid soldiers."

"Black Watch have the rep."

"They're good guys. Really respected me. Had my back."

"And you had theirs. I know that about you."

Not enough. We lost Mick.

Dumping my clothes into the machine, I think back to the grape hut. I can't get it out of my mind.

"You still sexting with that guy?"

"Yeah."

"That's good. A distraction."

We stand in silence for a while, listening to the swish of the machine. I pull a Coke can out of my pocket and hand it to him. A broad smile crosses his face. "Ah, you remembered! I missed you, Burns, but I also missed this."

He pops the can open and takes a long swig. "Want to watch Dane?"

Shrugging, I hand him my laptop, and we sit down in the hot sun. He presses "play" on the Dane Cook comedy album and starts to laugh within the first minute. I try to force a smile, but I can't and instead stare down at my feet, watch the swirling sand and think of Mick.

LAUGH

Come on, Kelsi.

Laugh.

Don't be such a downer.

Look at me, for instance.

I've been through shit myself, but I can still laugh at you.

You are falling apart at the seams, and it's hilarious!

Halfway through fire watch duty, another Canadian and I look for signs of the enemy. The sun has barely risen, but the heat is already uncomfortable. My partner doesn't talk much, which is fine by me. I just pace back and forth, gripping my rifle. As soon as it's over I will check if Brady messaged me, pop a sleeping pill, and try to get some rest.

I hear a faint moo and look to my right as Emma waves at me. I just stare at her without lifting my arms. Something's off. Narrowing my eyes, I can plainly see that she's there and she's waving, but shit— she has a weapon!

My machine gun is racked at my shoulder. I remember what they told me when I went out with the British: *Don't hesitate to fire.*

I put a round in the chamber and aim my weapon at her.

"Burns!" My fire watch partner rushes to my side. "What do you see?"

"That little girl down there has a gun."

"Where?"

"Right fucking there!"

Dust kicks up behind my boots as I race down to the coms tent. "There's a girl with a gun right outside the FOB. She's going to shoot us."

The coms guy radios my partner to confirm what I've seen, but his voice comes on the radio. "The girl is unarmed. Burns—"

I run out of the tower to the coms tent. At this point, I was done.

SEEING THINGS

What just happened, Kelsi?

You could have ended that innocent child's life.

You're a monster.

Is this why you joined the military? What would your mother say?

What will stop you from hurting someone when—if—you make it back home?

You're a menace to society and a danger to everyone.

"Burns, I need a Coke," ribs Gould as he and McMillin join me for GD (general duty) on the American side of the compound.

"Drink some damn water, ya rocket!"

He smirks and takes a drink. "The Brits are rubbing off on you, I see. How are you doing?"

"Fine."

"It would be okay if you weren't fine. You know that, right? Seeing what you saw out there isn't easy to bounce back from."

We're quiet for a while, watching the Afghan workers and quoting war movies. It's one of the many things I've incorporated into my routine after my week with the Brits.

One of the Canadians walks up, and with a smirk, says in French, "Burns, I heard what happened on your fire watch shift. You're seeing things now?"

"Fuck off."

"Easy there, Burns. You seem crankier than usual. On your period?"

There's nothing I'd rather do in this moment than take the butt of my rifle to his face. Instead, I let out a long sigh. "It happens when you've spent time outside the wire, but you wouldn't know about that, would you?"

This shuts him up, and he walks away.

Gould smirks. "Go, girl."

"You know the first thing he said to me when I got back was, 'You're all in one piece, there's not a scratch on you. Don't be such a pussy.'"

"Ignore them." Gould kicks at the sand. "They're jerks."

"And that other guy, he actually asked me, 'Did you have any witnesses?'" I take a long drink of water from my canteen. "Then he said, 'That's what happens when you send a woman to do a man's job.'"

"Don't even listen to them. You're as strong as any man here. Actually, you're stronger than a lot of them."

"Yeah, but they laugh behind my back. I know it. And they talk about me in French, knowing I don't always understand what they're saying."

"We'll take care of them on the baseball field," McMillin winks. For a moment, I smile and then look him straight in the eyes.

"They don't believe anything actually happened to me."

"Does that even matter?"

I shrug. "Everything just makes me so angry. The smallest thing."

"That's normal." McMillin leans in closer to the two of us. "Gould put his fist through a wall when we lost one of our buddies."

I look down at my feet for a while. "So did you guys ever wonder why?"

McMillin shifts his feet and takes a deep sigh. "You mean why them and not me?"

I nod.

Gould crushes the can with his fingers. "All the time. Still do."

"It never leaves you. You just learn to live with it." McMillin gestures to the French Canadians. "It's something they will never understand, but you're one of us now, Kelsi."

Gould doesn't skip a beat. "We've got your back."

I smile and turn to face them. "They won't understand that it's about the men next to you, and that's it. That's all it is."

Gould lifts a bottle of water. "*Black Hawk Down*, 2001."

Now that I'm back with the Americans, I don't miss the British guys quite so much. These men and I were not in a position, or in a pay grade, to understand what was fully going on in that war. But what we did understand is what we were told, and that what we were doing was right. We'll always have that, no matter how it all turned out. No matter that it looms larger in our minds than our futures, which seem to be unspooling before us at a rate we cannot control.

POOR KELSI

> Someone getting a little paranoid now?
>
> Perfect.
>
> Yes.
>
> Those French guys are just like the bullies in school, aren't they?
>
> The only way to get away from the bullies is to give in to me.

Weeks before the rest of my unit, I'm sent back to KAF, while the military tries to figure out what to do with me. I'm assigned to a special sort of hell called QM—the quartermaster. The quartermaster is a military officer who is responsible for providing quarters, rations, clothing, and other supplies. My job would be organizing and counting office supplies.

On the table in front of me there are thousands of pens, which I'm sorting according to color while rage oozes through my veins. I want to stab myself in the eye with one of these pens. Two weeks of busy work, and I am *done*. This is *not* why I joined the Army.

A colonel approaches me. "Burns, where's your magazine?" "Where's my ammo?" I snap back.

"Yes. The magazine you're *supposed* to have on you at *all* times at KAF."

"Actually, I have no *fucking* ammo left. I used it while shooting at people because I'm a *real* soldier."

The minute the words leave my mouth, I know I shouldn't have said them, but it's too late, and I can't take them back.

"You're done with QM, Burns. Get your ass to the shrink."

GOOD, KELSI

Things are going exactly as I hoped they would!

I'm seeing good things from you.

You're making excellent progress.

You're one step closer to being completely abandoned by the military.

Can't you sense it?

Oh, just you wait.

It's coming.

Discharged soldiers are my favorite.

Sergeant Leblond comes to KAF to see me. He's so upset, he's close to tears. "Kelsi, this is serious. They've started the paperwork. You verbally assaulted a CO!"

I stare at him blankly. "I know. I fucked up."

"You could end up on trial in the military courts. It happens all the time."

"I don't know what you want from me. I can't take it back."

"You have to give me something here. They're going to come after you, and they'd be totally within their rights to do so!"

His face is red, and the gravity of what's happening here starts to sink in.

I don't say anything.

"Kelsi, for Christ's sake, help me out here."

"What am I going to do?"

"Well, what did the doctor say?"

"That I have acute post-traumatic stress trauma."

"Okay. That's something. I'll start working on getting you a medical discharge."

"I don't want a discharge. I don't want to leave."

"Want to go to court instead? It's the only way to save yourself."

"Then what?"

He shakes his head. "This doesn't happen often, so I'm not sure exactly what's next. Just be ready to go in case you're cleared early."

"I want to finish my tour." I stare him down.

"I know you do, but you might not have a choice here."

"You need me on the guns. You said so yourself."

"I need you well."

I won't leave yet. I need to get revenge on the monsters who killed my friend.

FINISHED

The guys are laughing at you because

You're a JOKE.

You're weak.

You're "sick," but you don't look sick to me. Or to anyone.

You should be taught enough to get through this.

The others do it.

You should be able to block me out, you piece of shit.

You don't deserve to wear the uniform.

FIFTEEN

Released

August 2009

Sitting in front of a military doctor again, tapping my foot, I wait for him to give me more pills and tell me I'll be fine in a few weeks.

"Burns, I'm not seeing much improvement."

"Okay." I rub my hands together on my lap, my eyes darting around the room. "So what's wrong with me?"

"I think we're dealing with post-traumatic stress disorder."

"I thought that's what I already had?"

"We thought it was acute, but it isn't getting better. It's not going to go away on its own."

"So what happens now?"

"You'll be sent home."

"But I'm not finished with my tour."

"You aren't fit to serve, Burns."

"I'm fine."

"Are you sleeping better?"

"Yes." I lie because I don't want to go home.

"Is your appetite okay?"

161

I nod and sit on my hands to stop myself from wringing them. There is silence as he stares at me, and I try to pretend I'm okay. He opens and closes my folder, all the while looking back at me. I fear he can see through me.

Next, I'm sent to the major's office. I sink into his leather chair, feeling small and vulnerable. "Feeling okay, Burns?"

"Yes, Major."

"You ready to get back on the guns?"

Music to my ears. I sit up taller. "Absolutely."

He laughs and looks me straight in the eyes. "Well, there's no chance of that happening."

My heart sinks.

He opens my file and takes out the thick stack of paperwork. "All of this has been filed since your return from outside the wire."

He shoves it across the desk, and his face turns dark. "Severe PTSD?"

"That's what the doc says."

"Burns, you're more of a problem for me than anything."

My cheeks redden.

He stuffs the papers back into the folder and slams it on the desk. "There's nothing worse than a useless soldier."

I bite my lip and wring my hands.

"Frankly," he stands up, "it would have been better for me if you'd died."

Did he really just say that? My eyes sting as I try to hold back the tears.

"Less paperwork to deal with." He motions to the door. "Get out of here."

USELESS SOLDIER

Let that sink in for a minute; get good and comfortable with it.

"It would have been better if you died."

162

The sounds of a ball hockey game almost make me forget that I'm in Kandahar. Watson, whose tour is almost up, places a coffee in front of me and sits down at the table. "Careful not to burn your tongue."

I look at the dark circles under his eyes. "Not getting much sleep?"

He shakes his head. "You?"

"None." I pull the lid off the cup, releasing a cloud of steam. "How's Max doing?"

"Eh, haven't heard a thing, but he'll be all right. I miss the bastard."

"I miss everyone." I pause for a moment. "Including Mick."

We sit in silence for a bit, sipping our coffee. "Why..." I start and then stop. "Why wasn't it one of us?"

"I told ya, Burns, I'm set to go August 10th, and you September 10th. Hurry up and wait!"

I try to smile but can't.

Watson reaches out a hand. "It would be strange if you didn't wonder why it wasn't you. Why wasn't it any of us? It's just natural to think about it that way. Part of the problem with having a tactical mind is that you'll always think that if it were five minutes later or earlier it coulda been me. It's normal to go there."

"Yeah, I guess."

"How are you coping with it all? How are the Canadian arseholes behaving?"

"Just like I thought they would. They don't believe anything happened."

"Aye. You need to get your hands on some dead goats and put them in their tent."

"Great advice, thanks." I can't help but grin back at him. "I'm going to have to see a shrink."

"Braw. But keep talking to us. We were there with you. Just 'cause you're leaving here, that doesn't mean you're leaving the war. We've all still got your back."

"I guess so." I look down, then back up at Watson. "I'm sorry I'm leaving."

"You need the rest, Kels."

"I'll be back. I'll finish my tour."

"Aye, take care of yourself first. Where they sending you?"

"Back to Quebec. I'll get further instruction there."

"You'll be all right, Kelsi. You're strong. We all know it. We all know you're a lot tougher than any of those dobbers."

I laugh. I'm going to miss him. Being with these guys gives me a sense of comfort, but it also hurts. No way am I ready to leave. There's still a part of me in the Panjwai district, and I am not ready to go home, but that's what's happening. It's out of my control.

Later that day, the door of the Herc closes on my life in Afghanistan. As I watch the dusty earth below while we take off, I feel like I'm being taken from my family.

HOME

Hold the door.

I'm coming along to make sure the sights and sounds of Afghanistan never, ever leave you.

I'm the perfect souvenir.

When I land in Quebec, no one is there to pick me up, of course, because the rest of my unit is still in Afghanistan. But shouldn't someone be there? I've done my duty; I've given all I have to give. And the military can't even pick up a soldier from the airport? Shouldn't they extend this simplest of courtesies? I wonder, briefly, if they even remember that I exist. Then I put the thought out of my mind. I have other things to think about.

After three connecting flights, I'm exhausted—mentally, physically, and emotionally—and I pace in the empty airport in Quebec at 0200. What am I supposed to do now? I try recalling names of people I know in Quebec and remember one of the nicer officers at the regiment who didn't deploy.

I look up his number in my contacts and call him. "*Salut!* It's Burns."

"Burns? Where are you calling from?"

"The airport. I'm sorry to call in the middle of the night, but I need someone to pick me up and take me to the regiment."

He replies, "I'll be there as soon as I can."

"Thank you."

While I wait for him, I send Brady a text. *Back in Canada.*

It's been almost a year since we met, but despite the distance, we've kept in touch.

In another minute, there's a reply:

Where are you?

Quebec. Airport. Waiting for someone to pick me up.

How was your flight?

Long. zzz

We text each other until Brady has to go to sleep. Like a normal person.

NEVER

That relationship will never go anywhere.

You know that, right?

Someone like you can't be with someone like him.

He'll never put up with me.

You can only have one of us, and I'm not going anywhere.

By the way, where's that military family of yours now?

Oh, that's right.

You're a useless soldier.

In full uniform, I wait at the regiment for people to start showing up for the day. The clock has changed from 0400 to 0500 since I've been here, which was when I brushed my teeth and changed my clothes. With nothing else to do, I watch time go by, until finally, at 0630, the RSM (regimental sergeant major) walks into the regiment and waves me over to follow him to his office.

He's a tall, intimidating man with broad shoulders and a strong jaw. He's a super soldier—someone you can't help but look up to. He must have been through what I've been through. He must understand.

"Burns, you're being reposted to Ottawa, where you'll be closer to the hospital for treatment."

"Wait...what? Reposted? I'm no longer part of the 5RALC?"

"Not anymore. You leave tomorrow."

Shaking my head in disbelief, my cheeks burn. "The place that was my 'home' for almost a year? I'm being tossed out to the hospital now? Just like that?"

He looks up past me and then back down at the stack of papers on his desk. Never have I been one of them. I am a replaceable number in a group of people who never wanted me in the first place.

He closes my folder and pushes it aside on his desk. "Check in once you arrive and wait for your next instructions."

The words from my major echo in my ears: *It would have been better for me if you'd died.*

There's nobody to say goodbye to. There's nothing left here for me. Good riddance.

PTSD

I'm coming with you.

You've never been one of them, but you're with me now.

You belong to me.

SIXTEEN

Civilian

September 2009

Sipping on a coffee in the Tim Horton's parking lot after a seven-hour drive, I scroll through my messages until I find the last text from Brady, the one that says:

Message me when you're home.

Made it back to Campbellford, grabbing a coffee and will be at my parents place in a few minutes. chat later.

Setting down the phone, I start to reverse the truck and hear a notification. Putting the truck back in park, I check the text.

Message me anytime you need to, ok?

k. wishing their new house was ready by now. not looking forward to sleeping in the motorhome. Since there house burnt down they were in the middle of a rebuild.

Until I pull into my parents' driveway, the only thing on my mind is what seeing everyone will be like. I'm so numb. I feel dead inside. How am I going to pretend that I'm happy to be home?

Houch bounds to my truck, the first one to greet me, and I bend down to cuddle him. In another minute, Dillon's there with the biggest smile on his face, tossing me around. Then Mom and Dad. Without a word, they just hold me and cry.

"Hey, when did you guys become a bunch of crybabies?" I try to keep things light.

Mom wipes her tears and smiles. "We've been getting some advice from a doctor about how we can help you over the next couple of weeks, honey."

Dad smiles, feebly, from beneath the peak of his ball cap, and there's an ache in my chest as I wish I was the same little girl as when I saw them last. But I'm not, and I never will be again.

"Me and Dad and Dillon. We're here for you."

"Thanks, it's really nice of you to want to help me."

Dad grabs my bags, and we walk toward the trailer. I just want to wander into my room and hide, but there's no room here for me anymore. I think back to my little space at Ramrod with its fancy castle plywood walls. What I would give to be there right now. For a chance to get back on the guns. When I step inside the motorhome, I'm silently reprimanding myself for not taking the howitzer carving with me when I hear, "Surprise!"

I stand there shaking, unable to lift my arms, my body overwhelmed.

High-pitched screams rip me back to reality. Shit.

A bunch of friends swarm me, hugging me and laughing and chatting loudly. The smell of wine coolers, deodorant, and perfume— more sweetness than I've smelled in months—is totally overwhelming. Everything is pressing in on me, and my head feels full.

"We're so happy you're home, Kels!" my friend Michel squeals.

Mom looks so proud. "The girls are going to take you out tonight to celebrate you being home."

"This is a pretty terrible fucking idea," I say through gritted teeth.

Mom looks hurt, and now I hate myself for making her feel bad, but I can't help it. I have no filter.

Grabbing a beer, I twist off the cap and follow the girls out the door.

At the bar, I stand in a corner where I can keep an eye on everything. My head pounds from the bright lights and loud music, but I keep watching the crowd, looking for anything suspicious.

When I step forward, a girl bumps into me and spills beer on my shirt. "Watch where you're going!" I snap and instinctively scan the floor for garbage and anything that looks out of place. *Forget it, Kelsi. You're in Canada now.* But I can't help it. And when one of my friends puts her hand on my arm, I shove her away, aggressively. "Get your hands off of me."

"Kels! Easy!"

Hating myself, I storm off, straight to the bar, and slam my glass on the counter. "Can I have another beer, please? Some cow spilled mine."

Michel is beside me again. "Kelsi, are you sure you want another one?"

"What, are you my mother now?"

I shove a ten-dollar bill across the bar, swig my beer in two gulps, and stomp away.

SHAME ON YOU

Your *normal* parents and *normal* friends are trying to be nice to you, you asshole.

Show some gratitude.

Smile.

Oh, wait.

I have your feelings now, don't I?

I have them locked up in a special little box where you will never find them ever again.

Have another drink, because alcohol is perfect for you right now.

Ba ha ha ha ha!

One eyelid opens and scans the room; I'm back in the motorhome. My mouth is dry, and there's a queasiness in my stomach. How did I get here? Slowly, I lift my head off the pillow, and the minute I do, the throbbing in my brain makes me regret it. Must...find...Tylenol. I reach for my phone to check the time: 1500.

The moment I wander into the kitchen, Houch is at my heels. Rifling through the cupboards, I find some painkillers and swallow a couple down with a glass of water.

Houch whimpers at my feet. "Dammit, Houch. Get away from me!"

He retreats and cowers in the corner, and I bend down to stroke his soft head. "Sorry, buddy. Come on outside with me."

When I check my phone, there are missed texts from Brady, the last one being, *hope you got home ok.*

I reply *ya. hungover.*

Grabbing my Oakleys from the counter, I head out to the yard and stare at the woods behind the house. It's quiet here, and the thick blanket of trees is soothing to the eyes. For a moment, I think back to chopping firewood with Dad, and I almost smile. But then I'm right back in Afghanistan, hearing the attacks, the bombs. I put my hands over my ears, then jump. No helmet. We always need to wear our helmets, ever since a soldier got his head sliced open with an axe by the Taliban during a prayer circle.

Houch cocks his head and lies down at my feet. *Jesus. What if someone comes out of those woods? I don't have a weapon.*

"Mom," I yell. "Where's the axe?"

She looks up from the garden bed and drops her trowel. "Why?"

I stare at her with a blank face. I know the Taliban isn't going to come out of the woods right now, but I can't calm down.

Mom walks toward me, dropping her gloves along the way. "How long do you plan on sitting out there?"

"I just got here." I look down at my phone—1700? I've been staring at the woods for two hours?

Mom bends down to look me in the eye, but I turn away. She has no idea what happened to me over there. I can't tell her, because her strained face tells me she's living her own nightmare by having me back. I hate myself for doing this to her.

"Are you hungry?" she asks.

Ignoring her, I go back into the motorhome and crack open a cold beer to chase down some sleeping pills. Back in my bed, I fall asleep, fantasizing about killing myself, and not for the first time. I wake up two days later.

END IT

It's time, Kelsi.

What kind of life is this?

You can't sleep without the scene replaying in your mind.

It's never going to stop.

Every night when you close your eyes?

That fear you have?

It's always going to be here.

You're a useless soldier.

You're extra useless without your guns.

You won't sleep tonight.

Keep taking your pills, and we'll all pretend they'll make this better.

It was Mom's idea to pick up a few items at Walmart before I move into my apartment in Ottawa, but I'm too agitated. I've never been in this store, and every aisle we walk down, I'm looking over my shoulder, scanning the shelves, turning corners cautiously.

"Kels, do you want this?"

"Uh-huh," I say without even looking at what she's referring to. My eyes repeatedly scan the store for things that are out of place.

"Mom, I need to leave."

"Let's just get a few more towels." Her voice is chipper, matching the sunny day. Why can't I be the same? It's beautiful outside. I'm alive, and I *should* be happy.

"*Now*, Mom." It's triggering as hell in here, but she doesn't realize it. How could she?

TRIGGER

```
Where's your weapon, Burns?
Look over there—I see a burka.
Do you?
```

At the checkout, Mom passes items to the cashier, and I help to bag them, but I'm on edge. I need to leave. Right now. I'm anxiously fidgeting with my fingers and tugging at the hems of my shorts. From the corner of my left eye I notice a family; the woman is wearing a burka, and the man narrows his eyes when he looks at me.

Rage wells up. Immediately I'm back on guard duty for the FOB, the day the Afghan worker tried to fuck around. He could have killed us all. He could have been the same person that killed Mick!

I start screaming at them, "Don't you fucking look at me! I'm going to kill your whole family, you piece of shit!"

BRAVO

```
WHAT A DISPLAY THAT WAS!
Good luck living with yourself.
Will tonight be the night?
```

Mom's face closes in as she shuffles me away, leaving our items on the counter, apologizing to some people, looking away from others. In the car, she pulls me toward her, stroking my hair, but I feel a damp spot on my shoulder and a slight tremor from her chest. Her little girl is broken, and there's nothing she can do about it.

Never have I hated myself more in my entire life. That family didn't do anything wrong. They're here in Canada. I was in the war—they weren't. All I can think about is killing myself and making all of this go away.

YES

```
Now we're talking.

Yes.

Yes.

Yes.
```

A few weeks later, I attempt to go out in public, but with a friend as protection. Even in the parking lot, with people walking and cars pulling in and out, I can feel my stress levels rising.

"Hey, asshole, that was my spot!"

"No road rage at the mall!" Michel chirps from the passenger seat of my brand-new Ford Escape. "I still can't believe you bought this car."

Locking the doors with my key fob, she follows me as I storm into the plaza.

"I don't even know what a car like that costs."

"Forty-six grand, baby."

"Holy shit, Kelsi! That's like—university tuition."

"It's only money. The Army pays well. Tax-free plus danger pay! You should see the new dirt bike gear I got. It's sick."

"You're racing again?"

"Yeah. Well, I plan to. I have nothing else to do. Besides, there's this guy."

We wander into the mall, and I buy us coffees while Michel heads to a nearby store. I catch up to find her looking through a rack of sweaters, rubbing her hand over one.

"You like that?" I hand her a coffee.

"Yeah, it's beautiful." She holds it up. "It would look good on you."

I shake my head.

Michel puts the sweater back, but I stop her.

"I'll buy it for you."

"No, Kels, it's too much!"

"I want you to have it. Try it on."

"I don't need it. I'm just looking."

"I'm just going to buy it when you leave, so you might as well humor me."

"Only if you will at least crack a smile today."

"I don't know how to."

"What does that even mean?"

"I know it's weird, but it's not in me anymore. I can't smile." Michel lifts up my cheeks for a moment and chuckles, but it's not happening. I'm numb. I don't feel anything. "Look. I can't make myself happy, but I can make you happy. It's a start."

We walk to the counter with the sweater, and as the cashier rings it in, Michel asks, "Are you getting any help with that?"

"I'm seeing a shrink every week, if that's what you mean."

"When do you think you'll be going back to work?"

I shrug. "I haven't heard from the military yet. They're still trying to figure out what to do with me."

We continue shopping, and I buy every single thing my friend shows interest in. Five thousand dollars later, her smile makes me feel a little bit better.

EMPTY

Your friends think you're a real piece of work.

You're a shit to be around, but as long as you keep spending your war money on them, they'll pretend to tolerate you.

Don't kid yourself.

They don't care about you.

Only I do.

Darkness surrounds me as I run into the heat, choking on smoke. Mortar rounds whistle through the air and land at my feet. I can't stop running. They're after me.

"Burns!" Mick screams. "Help!"

"Mick!" Bullets whiz past my head. "I'm coming!"

The stench of charred flesh and hot brass hang heavy in the air. Mick is pinned beneath a pile of rubble next to a fully engulfed grape hut, but I can't get to him. Suddenly my feet won't move.

"Watson! Johnny! Help! It's Mick!" Nobody answers. "Burns, help me!" he cries.

I reach for his arm, but I can't...quite...get to him. "Someone help me!"

Mick howls like a wounded animal as the flames consume him and his body becomes a giant fireball.

I wake up in a cold sweat, screaming. My newly adopted orange tabby kitten, Tuck, bounds out of my bed and rushes from the room, his claws scraping the floor. My heart races, and I bury my head in my hands.

The clock glares at me with its red numbers, 0300. Within a minute or two, Tuck jumps back up and burrows under my blanket, scratching at the fabric. I pull him up to my chest and rub softly under his chin until he starts to purr. That rhythmic sound soothes me, and I close my eyes with the tickle of his whiskers and his rough tongue on my cheek.

"So far you're all that's saving me from myself, buddy." He looks at me lovingly through glowing amber eyes. "That's right. I can't die because you'll be all alone."

Tuck closes his eyes, and eventually I do too, trying to fall asleep. But then a roar from outside startles me, and Tuck jumps from the bed again. A weight on my chest stops me from sitting up.

"What was that?" I call into the night. Tuck meows, pacing back and forth in the doorway, his tail held high.

My head sinks back into the pillow. *Kelsi. Calm yourself. You live in Army housing now, by the airport. That was a plane.*

175

No matter how many deep breaths I take, I'm not calming down, and Tuck hasn't returned either.

I quickly do the math to figure out what time it is on the West Coast. Midnight. I punch in Brady's number.

A groggy voice answers. "Hey!"

"Brady? Did I wake you up?"

"Yes, but that's okay. Is this a booty call?"

"I had a really bad nightmare."

"Do you want to talk about it?"

"No, but can you distract me?"

"Are you naked?"

QUIT IT

Did you notice that he didn't really seem all that happy to hear from you?

You woke him up.

You're a weak child, and you are wasting his time.

This is never going to end between you and me.

Do it.

SEVENTEEN

Roo

October 2009

My suicide is all planned out, and I am at peace with the idea. My will was written before my deployment, and everything's in order. I know what I'm going to do, and it will happen tonight; but Brady keeps coming into my mind. Before I make my move, I want to call him and say thanks for being there. Tapping his numbers into the phone, I wonder what I'll say when his voicemail picks up. Should I tell him thank you? Or goodbye? Or both? He was, after all, the guy I imagined myself marrying. If he doesn't answer, that's a sign that I should just go ahead and get it over with now.

Instead, he picks up on the first ring. "Hey!"

Shit. I didn't think he'd answer, and his voice catches me off guard. "Oh, hey. You busy?"

"Just playing some pool with a couple of buddies. What's up? It's late there."

"Nothin.'"

"Kels, are you crying?"

I don't speak.

"Kels, what's wrong?"

"Oh, I'm fine. I just wanted to hear your voice, and ya know, to thank you for always being so easy to talk to."

"I'm here for you. You know that."

"Thanks."

After a minute of deafening silence, he says, "Hey, I'm going to be in Montreal next week. You're not far from there, right?"

"Um, no, just a couple hours' drive."

"Will you come see me?"

My heart starts to pound in my chest.

"Really?"

"Yeah, really. I want to see you. And other stuff."

"Okay."

"Promise?"

"Yeah, I'll come see you."

Shit. I'm committed. Now I have to stay alive.

"Can't wait!"

"Me too." Brady is holding me together. It might be with tape and string, but I am alive.

A MATTER OF TIME

All he wants is sex.

Actually, that's one of the things people try to use as a weapon against me.

Good luck with that.

October 2009

Standing outside the hotel door, I force a smile, the way I've been practicing, take a deep breath, and knock. I'm happy to finally see Brady, but a smile just isn't forming. My face doesn't know that expression anymore.

Brady opens the door, and without a word, pulls me in close, and for the first time in months, my brain goes still, focused only on this moment. He caresses my cheek as our lips meet, and I wrap my arms around him so tightly, all I feel is the beating of his heart against my body.

When we pull apart for air, he grins and leans back for a moment, studying my face. A smile is there, if only for a short moment. His hand drifts to my waist, and he leads me into the room. Our bodies entwine till there is no space between them, and I feel like I'm home. Everything we texted about doing together for the past year is more electrifying than I ever imagined.

Even during our last moment together, as I drive him to the airport in the morning, my worries are suspended as he rests his hand on my thigh. "Thanks for coming to see me."

"I had fun hanging out, partying, watching you race super cross!" I pause when I think of returning to regular life. The distance between Vancouver and Ottawa is far. "Hopefully we can see each other again soon."

"You'll have to come out to the West Coast."

"I love Vancouver. I was there once for Tae Kwon Do."

"Well then, we'll have to—"

I don't hear the rest of what Brady says. An older-model beige sedan merges into my lane, and my heart starts racing. There could be explosives in that car. The scent of clean dirt attacks my memory, and I feel the grit of sand in my teeth. I have to keep us safe.

Checking over my right shoulder, I step on the gas and swerve around the car, putting as much distance between it and me as possible, coming about an inch away from smashing into a concrete barrier.

"Shit, Kelsi. You're going to hit something!" Brady shouts.

I take a quick look over my left shoulder to make sure I'm clear.

"What the hell was that about?" Brady loosens his grip on the door.

For a minute, I don't know what he's talking about. We're safe. Then I see the fear on his face. "Oh, God, I'm sorry."

Brady puts his hand back on my leg. "You okay?"

"Yeah." How am I going to explain this without sounding crazy? "Those were the kind of cars they put bombs in over there. I'm sorry I freaked out."

"I get it. I can see how that would be a trigger. Want me to drive?"

"No. I'm okay. I'm sorry. I'm a crazy person."

"Hey, most girls are crazy. At least you have a good reason to be. If you came back from there and weren't a little messed up, I'd be worried."

For a single moment, time stops. He always knows the right thing to say. Careful, Brady Sheren. I might be falling for you.

CAREFUL

> It won't be any fun for me if you die in a car wreck!
>
> It's a good thing there aren't many old beige cars on the road these days.
>
> OH WAIT!
>
> Ha ha ha ha.
>
> Buckle up.

A week later, I'm walking among neon-lit resorts and twenty-four-hour casinos on the Las Vegas strip with Brady. He's racing, and I'm here to watch again, but it's turning out to be more than that. This is Vegas, after all!

As much as I love checking out the swanky hotels and the campy attractions, I can't stop looking over my shoulder. There are so many people who look like an enemy here, and the crowd is noisy. Always, I'm on guard, and even though Brady has my hand, my chest tightens.

If it weren't for being here with him, I would have left after the first night of walking among these hordes of people, but the only time I feel anything is when I'm with Brady. Since I last saw him, we've talked on the phone every day, we text continuously, and I can't get him out of my head.

We're looking in a display window when a whistle slides through the air and explodes with a loud bang. I collapse and curl into a fetal position, tears streaming.

"Shit! Kels?" Brady bends down to hold me. "It's okay. It's just fireworks."

Covering my ears, I continue to sob.

Gently, he pulls me up and away from the crowd. "You're okay," he whispers softly.

"I'm all fucked up." My voice cracks through my tears. "I'm so sorry."

"Don't apologize. I admire you."

"For what?" My voice wavers.

"You're so tough."

"Yeah, real tough." I wipe at my tears.

He motions to a group of girls walking by. "You're not concerned with trivial things like most people are. Breaking a nail, likes on Instagram; you let those silly things slide because it's not worth getting excited about. You're cool as hell."

FIREWORKS

So much for the fireworks between you and Brady.

Looks like that little problem will solve itself.

Some gunner you are.

Can't even handle the sound of fireworks.

You weak little child.

Let's play some more...

"Gould died." I read in a Facebook message.

"No." My stomach lurches, and I crumple to the floor. My breath, my heart, everything feels like it stopped with those words.

"I'm sorry, Burns. I know he meant a lot to you. He meant a lot to me, too," said McMillin

"What happened?" I want to cry, but tears won't come.

"He was inside a tank when it rolled over an IED."

"Jesus."

"Pressure from the blast caused his heart to burst. He stood up, said he wasn't feeling right, then sat down and fell asleep and died."

I hold on to this voice from my past and count the names of my other friends that are still fighting over there. "Thanks for messaging me."

I close the computer and let out a blood-curdling scream that echoes among the walls of my room. All I want is to go back there and get revenge on the people who built the IEDs that killed Mick and Gould.

I curl up in bed and wail.

My phone vibrates again. When I see Brady's name flash across the screen, I hesitate for a second before picking up. "Hi, Brady."

"Hey, Kels, what's going on today?"

I can't speak.

"Everything okay?"

"No..." I want to feel sadder. I want to be able to cry for Gould. "I wish you were here..."

"What is it?"

"Gould is dead."

"Ah, shit, Kels, I'm sorry. He's the Coke guy, right?"

"Yeah. Such a good guy."

"Tell me about him."

"We did laundry together once a week, and then we'd watch the Dane Cook show. He helped me get through those awful days when the guys in my unit were such assholes. War sucks."

"I know." His gentle voice soothes me.

"He helped me keep it together when I came back from my op." I pause for a moment. "He was always there when I needed someone to talk to. Like you are now."

I'm quiet for a minute, but Brady stays right there, listening. He's the only bright spot in my life, but even though we're officially dating now, I don't feel I deserve him.

"He's so young. Now his parents have to bury their beautiful, gentle son, and I didn't get to say goodbye. I didn't get to thank him."

"I'm sure he knows that he meant a lot to you. You don't exactly hide your emotions!"

I laugh nervously for a moment and then grow silent again.

"Do you think you'll get some sleep tonight?"

"No."

"Try."

"Other than when I'm with you, I haven't had a good sleep since before I deployed."

* * *

Gould sits beside me in his full kit. He doesn't say a word but reaches into his pocket and pulls out a can of Coke. He pops it open, raises his hand to toast, and smiles at me. Then, he's gone.

I sit up in bed wringing my hands, wrapping my soaked sheets around me. Gould came in a dream to say goodbye.

Through my tears I whisper, "I will never forget you, Gould. I'm thankful for the time I got to know you and call you my friend. See you in Valhalla."

LIGHTS OUT

```
You're hanging on longer than I expected.
How much longer can you keep this up?
Such stamina.
I'll have to try harder.
```

EIGHTEEN

Restart

January 2010

After being home for four months, following the military diagnosis of post-traumatic stress disorder, I finally hear from my employer. Four months of stress and anxiety, four months of depression, four months of contemplating suicide on a daily basis.

Now I'm being posted to cleanup duty at a range in Ottawa used by RCMP (Royal Canadian Mounted Police), military, special forces, and for competitive shooting. My job will be to clear the range after it's been used and make sure that conservation rules are being followed in the sanctuary. If this works, I can be retrained and keep serving.

I work from 0700 to 1300 two days a week, and eventually my brain adjusts to the sound of rounds going off all day long. Several months into the job, a coworker and I drive out to clear the range after a course. We walk along the cushiony green grass, about fifty meters or so, to a sandy spot where everything lands after being thrown. Gould's sunglasses shield my eyes from the late August sun, which in Ottawa is frosty compared to Afghanistan. I think back to the first time I ever held a grenade in my hands, and at this moment, I wish I was shooting instead of cleaning up after them. I feel like a failure that I couldn't finish my tour.

Sand.

Blistering heat.

Sun.

The intoxicating scent of gunpowder.

Just before the sand, I collapse. Tears pour down my face, and I gasp for breath. I can't move. I'm completely frozen. Why Mick and not me or the others?

"You okay, Burns?"

All I can do is shake my head. I am paralyzed by fear and can't understand why.

"It's okay. Take a minute. Just breathe." Gently, he helps me back to my feet.

SANDBOX

Remember the sand that poured out of your braid and your boots after you got back from Op Herrick?

You're welcome.

Before long, I'm meeting with my case manager, who tells me without any emotion or thanks, "We believe you can no longer do your job effectively. You're being medically released from the Army." My eyes well up as I look at her from across the desk.

"But—I love my career. I love the Army. Don't take away the only thing I'm good at. Please!"

She looks away from me and shoves the papers across the desk. "You'll need to sign the paperwork to start the discharge process."

"What else am I going to do? I have nothing! I dropped out of college."

She looks right through me. "You'll also need to turn in your kit."

Some other kid is going to get my equipment. The helmet that stopped shrapnel from piercing my brain, the webbing that's still stained with Mick's blood (they said they would destroy it but didn't), the sleeping bag that was my sanctuary during war, the shirt that caught my tears when I watched another human blow up in a million pieces, the rifle that saved my life and others, the vest that held the bulletproof plates that protected me from the Taliban's rounds. Every piece of my clothing with my name painstakingly stitched inside will be washed, stripped of my identity, and assigned to someone else.

My life is being turned in to the next number, to the person who will take my place. I can almost hear my heart breaking. Then it hits me. "Where's my medal?" It would take me two years to get my General Campaign Star.

"Your unit has it. You'll get it when you get it."

And with that, she gets up from her desk and ushers me out the door.

I don't want to leave the Army, but I am not allowed to stay.

NUMBER

What?

You thought they would reward you for something?

What good did you do?

You freaked out, had a little meltdown, and got sent home like the baby you are.

Hot brass falls down like rain. Bullets whiz past my head. My weapon is on the dirt a meter ahead of me, but my boots won't budge. I'm frozen. An Afghan worker charges at me, wielding an axe, and I'm paralyzed. I scream, but no sound comes out of my mouth.

I feel lips on my face. "Wake up, Kels," Brady whispers in my ear. "You're having a bad dream. It's okay."

My mouth is dry, but my skin is drenched in sweat and tears. Brady wraps me in his arms and gently strokes my hair.

"Was that a bad one?"

"Uh-huh." I try to catch my breath.

"You were kicking this time, along with the twitching and mumbling." He kisses my forehead.

"I'm sorry I woke you up."

"Shh, no apologizing."

After a second or two, I realize what day it is and that I'm in Vancouver with Brady and his family. I whisper, "Merry Christmas!"

Brady pulls me so close that there's no space between us; we fit together perfectly. "You're the best Christmas gift I could ever ask for."

Other than visits with Brady, the year has been a blur, with me in a drug-induced fog. Hospital for treatment, working through triggers, motocross racing, and time at the gym. After the gifts have been opened, we sit back, admiring the lights on the Christmas tree: Brady, his gentle-hearted sister Nessy with tattoos decorating her arms, his youthful parents, Rick and Shelley, and me.

Rick and Shelley sit next to each other. I'm curled up on Brady's lap, as usual, and it feels like I'm in a scene from a Christmas movie.

"You two are like a couple of kangaroos." A smile crosses Rick's kind face. "Always stuck together."

We laugh but can't deny it. Brady pulls me closer, and I love how his arms feel around me. And the warmth of his body behind me. I feel safe here. I love it here. "You're my kangaroo," Brady says.

"You're my Roo, too."

"It's so lovely having you here, Kelsi." Shelley lifts a gift from the floor, her toned biceps bulging.

"Thanks." I snuggle closer to Brady, his chin resting on my shoulder. "I love being here."

"Do you have your release date yet?" Rick's hand brushes his goatee.

"May 23rd."

"What then?"

"I'm not exactly sure." I look at Brady. "But I'd like to come back out here."

"We're thinking of getting a place together." Brady squeezes my hand.

"Oh, that's silly," Shelley says, her eyes sparkling. "You should come here and stay with us. There's plenty of room. Save your money for a down payment."

"Really?" I can't believe they could be so lovely to me. They barely know me.

"Of course. You're family."

HMMM

You're attaching yourself to more people.

Excellent.

Now you have more people to disappoint!

This will make my job a little bit easier.

The self-loathing should step up a notch now as you realize you're not worthy of love.

My snore wakes me. Then the pounding starts, a vice grip on my head. Reaching out my left hand, I feel the cold tile floor. Am I in the bathroom? I open one eye and look to my right. Tuck is licking the peanut butter off a butter knife I'm still holding in my hand. What the hell? I push myself off of the floor and lean against the wall. My head pounds, but I force my eyes to open again. Tuck is nuzzling my hand, and I scratch his back to stop while squinting at the oven clock: 3:15 a.m.

"Kels?"

"Yeah."

Nothing. Maybe he fell back asleep.

"Roo?" It's louder now. His feet hit the floor above me. Shit! I pull the half a loaf of bread from the counter and stick it in the fridge. The lid for the peanut butter jar is on the floor. How much of this did I eat? I fumble with it and then shove it into the cupboard half-closed.

"Kels?" Brady's running down the stairs now and into the hallway. I step into the light, holding on to the counter. He's standing there, my T-shirt in his hands, the pill box in the other. The evidence says it all, and I look down at my feet, anywhere but into the eyes of the man who has done everything to pull me out of this darkness.

"Babe..." His voice is tender and kind. Always is. I bite my lip to fight back a tear. I've scared him again. I'm an asshole, and I don't deserve him.

My legs buckle, and I slide down the wall to the floor. Brady brushes hair from my cheek and then scans my eyes with concern. His strong hands cup my chin. *You are always there.* I force a smile, and relief spreads across his gorgeous face. I reach out to his hands but hold on to thin air. Wait. I rub my blurry eyes. This isn't Brady's kitchen. I'm in Ottawa, not Vancouver.

I'm losing it.

I pick up the butter knife and put it on the counter, then scoop Tuck into my arms, making my way through the fog back to my bed, wishing Brady were here to tell me everything will be okay. I need to be with him like I need oxygen. I can't breathe without him.

* * *

After six months, the paperwork has been processed, and I open the letter from the Department of Veterans Affairs Canada that says *Thank you for your service....*

My nostrils flare as I take a deep breath, thinking about how they have completely abandoned me.

Wish to inform you...

After all this.

...a 3b Medical Release as you have been deemed mentally unable to serve the Canadian Military.

Sitting down, I try to absorb the weight of these words.

I am a pensioned veteran at twenty-one years of age.

As I read the letter, I ask myself: If I knew what would happen to me, would I have still joined the Army?

My mind answers the question immediately: I would never want anyone to go through this, but I also wouldn't have done it any other way.

That's my mind, the mind of a soldier. Forever. For better or worse.

The next day, I'm on a plane heading west to British Columbia, where I will move in with Brady's family.

If I relocate my life there, maybe it will help me find the light.

SEE YOU THERE

How are those *pills* working?

Am I quieter now?

Have you found *peace*? Peace.

Pieces.

Pieces of *Mick* in the walls, on the floor, in your pockets.

You won't have quiet from me, no matter how many pills you take, so why don't you *stop*?

I'm collecting *soldiers*.

Twenty-two a day is my goal.

You're on my list.

Stop fighting me, because I won't stop.

Stop *listening* to Brady, because my voice is louder.

I want you more than he does.

He's going to *leave* you anyway, you *weak* pain in the ass.

Look, he's cleaning up your mess again.

When will you *give in*?

You can run, but you can't hide.

NINETEEN

An Invisible Injury

"Remember the first time you brought me here?" I tilt my head to lick a drip of chocolate peanut butter ice cream from the edge of my cone.

"To White Rock? Very well. It was our first official date." Brady squeezes my hand tighter as we stroll to the pier to watch the sun set over the Pacific.

A few people walk the beach like us, and others jog along the water's edge. We pass a family packing up shovels and a picnic basket; the dad shakes sand out of a blanket as the mom puts shoes on a crying toddler.

The child's wail echoes in my ears. I pull my chin to my chest as a scene from Afghanistan plays in my mind where I patted down babies, searching around their blankets and outside their diapers for money and drugs. I've made a child cry. I've scared them, even though that was the last thing I wanted to do. Some part of me can't believe I had to search the babies. They were innocents. Out of all of us there in that desert, they were the only innocent ones. But it was war. It strips everything down to the raw, and you can't give anyone the benefit of the doubt. Those measures were our survival.

"Kels?" Brady's hands are on my elbows. "You okay?"

I nod and look down at the ice cream dripping onto my shoes.

"You sure?"

"Uh-huh."

"Wanna talk about it?"

"No." I look away for a moment, focusing on the shops and restaurants, the train tracks, people fishing on the pier, anything to distance myself from Afghanistan.

"Wanna go?" He places his hand gently on my shoulder.

"No, let's walk some more. I'm fine."

"Okay." He pulls me close, and despite the heaviness in my chest, I feel warmth return to my body. I love this little beach community, the ice cream, the water, but I'm detached from everything. I feel as emotional as a robot.

"You always seem to know when something is bothering me." I step onto the pier and heave a big sigh.

"I'm getting to understand you." Brady leans against the railing. "You're normally chatty, so when you get quiet, I know something's wrong."

The tide is coming in, and I watch the water collecting in little pools. I didn't notice when I went quiet or that my ice cream melted down my hand. I just go off into this other world as if everything around me is a void.

Brady runs his fingers over my forehead. "See, and then your eyebrows go down, and you make this squinty forehead face." He smiles and entwines our fingers. We stand there for a long time, watching the water creep back in. When I'm next to him, my thoughts and worries disappear.

"Ya know, ice cream *used* to make me happy. But I can't *feel* happy anymore."

"What else made you feel happy?"

I gaze out at the pier lights reflecting on the calm surface of the water. "The beach made me happy. Motocross made me happy." I turn to him. "The closest thing I feel to happy now is being with you."

Brady drops my hand and puts his arm around me. "I bet the doctors at the Operational Stress Injury clinic will be able to help you."

My chest rises and falls with a big sigh. "I hope so, Roo. I really hope so."

"How are you feeling about your appointment?"

I start pacing with just the thought. All I want is for my life to become normal, and I grab Brady's hand to hold on to the good things in my life.

"Like the last thing I want to do is open up to strangers about my story." My stride quickens the more I talk. "It's a trust thing."

"Want me to go with you?"

His pace matches mine step for step. "Yeah. Maybe just to wait with me?"

"Whatever you need."

I stop walking and turn to face him. My fingers lace behind his head, and he wraps his arms around me, picking me up off the ground. His lips find mine as the sun sets behind us. The only thing that would make this moment any more perfect is if I could feel some sort of emotion for this man who is everything to me.

* * *

After ten minutes of small talk, Dr. Greg Passey scratches his mottled goatee and says, "So, Kelsi, I've been asked to make recommendations about your meds. Can you tell me what you're currently taking?"

"Oh, yeah, sure." I reach into my purse and root around, the pill bottles rattling. "I brought them all because I can never remember the names."

I plunk ten bottles on the desk and check his face for judgment, but I don't see any. Instead, his deep-set eyes scrutinize every bottle, turning them over, reading the labels, and making notes. I've been through so many rounds of medications that I'm wary of taking anything different, let alone from a new treatment doctor, but this guy comes highly recommended.

I run my fingers along the soft arm of the leather couch and look around his small office. Framed certificates hang on the bone-colored walls, and potted plants brighten rows of books.

"It's common for someone with PTSD as severe as yours to be on this many medications." Light reflects off the top off his bald head as he tilts his face upward. "But let's try prescribing something that will be easier for your body to handle."

"Okay." I can't stop wringing my hands, so I scan the room for something to lock in on. I wish the fish tank from his waiting room was in here, but instead, I look at his leather shoes. Perfectly polished. Can he possibly relate to what I went through? I haven't told anyone about Mick since it first happened, and I don't know if I can find the words. The story plays behind my eyes every minute of every day, and that's enough to deal with. Discussing it with someone else is going to be hard, and I'm scared of opening up to him.

"We've come a long way in understanding Operational Stress Injury, or more commonly known as PTSD, since Iraq." Dr. Passey settles back in his chair. "That means veterans like yourself, from Afghanistan, and those from Desert Storm, have a bit of an advantage. There's a lot more research and better medications, but it's still going to be a lot of trial and error to see what works best for you."

I nod, relieved that he's doing the talking, but as I lean back, my foot still shakes.

"How much do you understand about PTSD, Kelsi?"

I shrug. "It's fucked me up and put me in a career-ending dark hole of hell. Beyond that, not much." I look out the window to break his gaze, Vancouver's skyline right in front of me. This is such a far cry from the hot, dusty world of Afghanistan. How could he begin to identify with what I experienced?

"PTSD would have been called shell shock in World War II or Vietnam," he says, pushing my half-inch-thick medical file to the side. The sun catches the silver glint of a duck on his window sill, and my eyes settle on it for a moment. Shiny and matte. Tough and fragile. In some ways, it reflects the two sides of me, PTSD and my old self. He stands up, looming over the bookshelf, and reaches for a photo. "I served for twenty-two years and have my own struggles with PTSD, so I know what you're dealing with."

"You're a vet?"

He nods and hands me a photo. "I was on many tours, including in Bosnia and in Rwanda."

So this guy gets me. He knows what I've been through.

"In the military, we are trained to disregard how we feel and to focus on the mission. I suspect you were very good at that."

I nod.

"What happened when you were over there was that a connection in your brain was severely injured, so communications aren't getting through properly. Your lower brain experiences a lot of anger, and it's trying to tell you something, but the connector to your upper brain is broken, so the message isn't being conveyed. All you know is that you're angry."

I look at him and nervously squeeze my hands together. "You mean it's an actual injury?"

"Yes, very much so."

"I'm not just crazy?"

"You're not just crazy," he reassures me in a calm, soothing voice.

"It sounds awful." I look down, then back at him. "But If I lost a leg or an arm in the war, people wouldn't ask why I was sent home with an injury when I look fine."

He listens as if he has all the time in the world and nothing is more important than my words. "It's tough coming home with an invisible injury, but we're going to adjust your medications and try some different therapies till we find something that works for you."

"I just want to start feeling again."

"My colleague, Dr. Mok, is going to join us now, and we'll talk about your triggers and help you understand your PTSD so you can start feeling better." There's a kindness in his voice that is so reassuring. "He and I will be your treatment team as long as you need us."

Dr. Mok walks into the office with a warm smile. "Hi, Kelsi." He takes a seat. "Let's talk about the symptoms you're experiencing."

"Well…" I pull at the sleeves of my sweater. "I don't sleep much, and when I do, I have horrible nightmares."

"Does it take you a long time to fall asleep?"

"Yeah. Usually at least forty-five minutes or an hour."

"And what are your nightmares about?"

"Always death and disaster. I wake up screaming sometimes, in a cold sweat."

Dr. Passey nods knowingly. "Do you have flashbacks?"

"A lot. I zone out when people are talking to me. I struggle in public places. I don't like crowds. I don't want to leave the house because when I see people who look like the enemy, I yell at them." I stop to catch my breath. "I know that it's not right for me to feel this way, but I can't do anything about it. Once you're trained to look for the enemy, you see them everywhere." I look down at my shoes for a long while, then back up at him. "It's like you carry the dead with you. That's the problem when you live."

"I understand," he says softly.

"I should have done more. It was mine and the others job to protect Mick."

"You couldn't have done more."

"Why did IEDs kill him and Gould? Why did I get within inches of taking a bullet to my hip? Why am I able to stop right before I kill myself?" I shake my head. "I just don't get it. Why do I deserve to be here?"

The moment my eyes widen, Dr. Passey furrows his brow in concern. "You're talking about survivor's guilt. Lots of veterans have it. I did."

For an hour or more we talk about my fears and my nightmares. For the first time, I feel that someone understands the cages of my mind.

At the end of my session, I'm exhausted but hopeful.

When I enter the waiting room, Brady walks over to us with a big smile and shakes hands with the doctor. His bright and happy nature is the kind of energy I need right now.

I'm silent as we walk out the door, and eventually Brady asks, "So, how'd it go?"

"Good. Dr. Passey's a vet. He gets me."

"Then you'll be going back?"

"Next week." I lean into him. "Thanks for being here."

He wraps an arm around my shoulder and snickers. "There were good candies in the waiting room!"

I pass the keys to Brady. "I'm so drained, I don't think I should be behind the wheel."

He rubs my arm and smirks at me. "You should never shrink and drive."

I slump into the passenger seat with a soft chuckle. Only Brady can make me smile like that.

CRAZY

I heard you talking about me, Kelsi.

I know Greg Passey very intimately.

I met him many years ago, and, well, he and I aren't big fans of one another.

But I do keep him in a job, so he should be more grateful than he is.

Anyway, you keep seeing him.

He's really only going to delay the inevitable.

I know you aren't going to be able to live with me forever.

I can wait.

TWENTY

Stuck

March 2013

I wake to pressure on my chest and fluff in my face as Tuck runs his rough tongue through my hair. "All right, all right." I stretch out my arms and yawn. "I'm up."

It's 10:30 a.m. I've slept in again. I rub Tuck's head as I sit up and put my feet on the cool wood floor. "I hope Brady fed you when he left for work." After Brady retired at age twenty from being a professional Supercross racer, he started a neck-brace safety company that helps prevent people from being paralyzed. Atlas Neck Brace Technologies.

My feet slide into fuzzy gray slippers, and I pull a hoodie over my T-shirt. I don't bother opening the blinds. Since I'm not going anywhere, it doesn't matter what it looks like outside. For three days following my last session with Dr. Passey and Dr. Mok, I've been in bed. Sharing my story broke me. A message from Brady is the only thing I look at on my phone:

Tried to get you up to join me for a walk this morning, but you wouldn't budge. Hope you have a good day.

Tuck meows, racing to his dish and back to me.

Sorry, Roo, I reply, *maybe we can go for a ride after you get home?*

I plod after Tuck and scoop a cup of kibble into his bowl. In his habitual style, he knocks the food onto the floor, nosing his way through it. "You're a weird cat, you know that?"

I turn to the fridge, and reaching past the fresh fruits and veggies, yogurt and milk, meat and eggs, I grab the leftover pepperoni pizza. Slice in hand, I pour a mug of coffee that Brady made and pop it in the microwave.

Crumbs from the pizza fall on the counter, and I wipe them off, scrubbing the surface like I cleaned everything last night. The house is spotless, and there is nowhere I can burn off any of this nervous energy.

I move to the couch, pulling a blanket over my bare legs, cupping the warm mug of coffee. Tuck crunches through his food, and I gaze at the wall.

Stare.

That's all I do these days, look absentmindedly at nothing.

The sound of the door opening breaks my trance. Tuck is curled up at my feet. "Hey, Roo? That you? You're home early." I take a sip of coffee to find it's ice cold.

Brady sits down on the couch beside me and gives me a kiss. "No, I'm not."

I pick up my phone to check the time: five o'clock.

"What did you do today?"

"Well, I got out of bed." Brady sits closer to me, and I snuggle into him. "I've been here on the couch ever since."

"You didn't go back to bed, so that's progress."

"I've been seeing Dr. Passey and Dr. Mok for months now. How messed up am I? Why am I not getting any better?"

"It's going to take time. You've been through a lot. It's okay."

"That's why I was nervous moving out of Rick and Shelley's house."

"Kels, we couldn't live with my parents forever. The plan was always for us to get our own place."

"I know, but it's so quiet here, and I have too much time to think. Shelley was always doing things with me that were distracting, and I miss working out with her." I start wringing my hands. "Besides, I love them."

"Wanna go for a run?" A mischievous grin crosses his face. "Or do other things to burn off some energy?" His breath is warm on my neck, sending goosebumps all over my skin as my knees go weak.

USELESS

What an outstanding contribution you're making to society these days.

Soon you'll break.

It's a matter of time.

As part of my exposure therapy, I'm maneuvering a shopping cart through the produce aisle, immersing myself in one of my most triggering environments. It's crowds that agitate me, but so far I've successfully filled half my cart. A man reaches past me, pulling a head of broccoli from the shelf. "Excuse me," I say, pushing out of the way, cutting off a woman pushing a cart laden with packaged foods. "Sorry!"

Guiding my cart quickly through the aisle, dodging other shoppers, I scan the store, trying to focus on my grocery list and not on the sound of babies crying. My lifeline, Brady, is sitting in the car waiting for me. All I have to do is buy the items on this list and get them to the car. I can do this.

Carrots. I put a bunch of them in my cart next to a container of salad greens. At the end of the aisle, I turn the corner to the dairy section. A simple pause to check my list, and my heart rate quickens. No matter how I try to regulate my breathing, it's still constricted and shallow. I take a deep breath and steer my cart straight to the yogurt section—I'm on a mission. As I face the wall of options and reach for Brady's favorite, in my peripheral vision, I spot a man in a turban.

I drop the container, and my fingers curl into a fist until I'm pinching my skin. I hear Max screaming, *Where's Mick?*

I take a step toward the man, but all the reasons not to do this come flooding in. I can't be here. I can't breathe.

Leaving my cart where it is, I pull my purse close to my body, turn around, and rush out of the store.

CLEAN-UP ON AISLE FOUR

```
That was so much fun!
I love exposure therapy.
Don't you?
Let's keep doing it forever.
The longer you keep at it, the sooner forever
will come.
```

My hands sweat as I rub the crinkled edges of the papers in my hand. I try to read the words that I wrote, but my eyes won't focus on them.

"It's all right, Kelsi," Dr. Mok reassures me. "Take a break."

"It's just," I start, curling my notes into a roll, "I can't do this now. I can't read about the things I did over there today."

"Maybe we've done enough exposure therapy." He scratches notes on my file.

"Yes, please. After all this time, I think it's only making things worse. There are too many triggers. Every time I go out in public alone, I panic. I can't get out of bed in the morning, and when I do get up, I have flashbacks constantly. If I actually manage to sleep, I wake up soaking wet from sweating, and I'm scaring the hell out of Brady every night."

"There are other therapies we could try. Some of our patients are having good results using medical marijuana."

"Not interested in cannabis, thanks."

"And is there a reason why you aren't interested?"

"There's too much stigma. Are there other options?"

He makes a note of this. "We can try some different things. But first, I think what would benefit you most is finding a purpose again. What's something you enjoy doing?"

I think for a minute. "Brady's been riding a dirt bike for fun since he retired from racing. I used to really like riding. Maybe I should get into it again."

"It's worth exploring," Dr. Mok says.

"I think the major was right. It would have been better if I died."

"Kelsi, you know that's not true. Don't you? Do we need to talk about that some more?"

"No, I'm sick of talking."

"One day you'll be able to actually go out and talk to people. You know that? One day you won't feel so raw."

I feel like he's lying to me, but I've never wanted to believe anyone quite so badly.

MOK'S WRONG

```
That doctor doesn't know anything.
You shouldn't believe him.
You're never going to be better.
Not until it's all over.
```

Adrenaline surges through me as I maneuver the dirt bike around the track, practicing with the guys before the race.

Approaching the face of a jump, I lift my butt slightly up off the seat, soften my knees, and give the bike a touch more gas when another rider crosses over into my lane. My leg goes out, and I land the bike with my foot off the peg. I feel the pop right away, and a burning sensation rips through my entire leg. Brady rushes over as I drag myself off the track, calling to me over the *brraaap* of the bike motors. "You okay, Kels?"

I dig my hand into the dirt for leverage and try to get up but can't manage to stand. "There's no way I can put any weight on my heel." I wince as I try once more. "I think I messed up my knee."

Brady helps me up, and I use him as a crutch to get to the car. "I told you you're a sketchy rider!"

"Not now, it hurts." I flinch with every step.

"I know, sorry. Let's get you to the hospital and see how badly you've injured yourself."

By the time we reach the hospital, my knee is swollen and discolored. "This one's going to hurt," the X-ray tech warns, twisting my leg in a position that sends a chill from my foot to my thigh. My nostrils flare.

"Ouch!"

"I know, but try to hold that there for one second." She gently sets the protective lead blanket over me, positions her camera over the top of my knee, and rushes back to take the image.

I grit my teeth and breathe.

"There." She pulls the lead blanket off, and I move my leg into a more tolerable position.

After three painful angles, we return to the emergency room, and each bed is full. The wait is long, but when the doctor projects the X-rays onto the screen, it's quite clear I've done some damage. "You can see here that you've injured your ACL." He points to the parts of my knee he's referring to.

"Jesus, it looks like I tore it in half."

"You require surgery, and unfortunately, one that isn't covered under your provincial health plan."

"When can I have it done?" I look to Brady. "I have enough left from my tour to pay for it."

The doctor waves over a nurse. "You'll likely need to wait for a couple of months for an opening, but we'll get you a date." He looks at me seriously. "Between now and then, and following the surgery, you won't be able to put any weight on that knee."

I sigh and look up at Brady's watchful eyes. "So much for finding meaning. I'll be right back where I was before—too much time on my hands to think."

"We'll get through it, Roo."

I'M HERE FOR YOU

> Ha.
>
> You thought a dirt bike would save you from me?
>
> You idiot.

Mom helps me fold laundry while we watch daytime talk shows on TV. "I appreciate you and Dad coming out here to help me. I know it's not easy taking time off from the rig."

"Well, it's been six months since your surgery. It's the least we could do."

I carefully place my jeans on top of the pile, smoothing out the creases, and cringe, noticing that the corners of Mom's towels aren't lining up. They would never pass inspection.

"Everything okay?" Mom points at the laundry basket that I'm staring at.

How long have I been zoned out?

"Do you need another painkiller, Kels?"

"I'm fine."

She adds a towel to the stack, her face lacking its usual liveliness. "It's been a long recovery time for you."

I sigh. "This has been a tough year. I can't really leave the house anyway, even if it weren't for my knee. I go as far as Dr. Passey and Dr. Mok's office for therapy and home again. That's pretty much it."

She musters up a stiff smile as she folds a towel. "Well, soon all of this will be behind you."

"It doesn't work like that, Mom." I get so sick and tired of explaining how I wake to this broken brain every morning and can't do anything else. Sleep, when it comes, is my only rescue. And now with this knee, it's even worse. I feel like I've taken ten steps backward for any gain that I've made.

"Oh, remember how you did Tae Kwon Do with a broken foot? You'll be back before you know it."

"I'm not a teenager, Mom. My life is different now."

"But you won't be like this forever."

My face heats up with suppressed anger, and my fingernails slice into my palms. I take a few deep breaths and release my grip slightly. "Mom, this is me now," I say through my gritted teeth. "This *is* how I am."

Dad calls from the other room, "Kelsi, your mother is just trying to help. Don't give her a hard time."

"We just miss that smile, Kels." Mom's face closes in. "That's all."

I plaster the biggest fake smile I can muster on my face, staring at her, wild-eyed. "There!" I say curtly. "How's this?"

Mom's shoulders drop. "Please, Kelsi, don't be like that."

If I didn't need help standing up, I would storm out of here, but just as I grab my cane and push myself off of the couch, Brady comes in.

"Hey, Roo, think we should go out and maybe get some fresh air?"

"That sounds like a great idea." Mom jumps up. "I'll start dinner. I thought I'd make some pork chops."

I stop in the hallway and grab my coat. "Mom! You know I can't eat pork anymore. It smells like—" I stop myself from finishing my sentence.

"Oh, don't be silly, you love pork chops."

"Thanks a lot, Mom." I turn my head away, holding back the tears. "Thanks for showing me how understanding you are."

As soon as I shut the door, I want to go back inside and apologize. But I can't. My mind snapped, and the anger is still growing. I want her to know that I wouldn't be here today if it weren't for her and Dad showing me how to be a strong person. Thing is, *I will* never be the same. This part of me can't melt away, and I'll never be who they want me to be. But I can't tell her that right now; I have to cool down and release my emotions into the darkness as I walk. And even that is hard.

After walking for a few minutes, Brady says, "You okay, Kels?"

"That's a loaded question." I tighten my grip on his hand as I limp along with my cane.

"Let's start with what I just saw there with your mom. You were pretty angry."

I take a deep breath as I shuffle down the sidewalk. "I am happy to have them here, but I'm just exhausted trying to pretend I'm normal. If I could walk, I would have left the room to keep the peace."

"They're trying." He lets out a big sigh.

"I know. We talk on the phone every day, but they don't know me anymore. Not this version of me. I feel like it's poison for them to see me like this."

"They love you no matter what."

"Yeah, but when I lose it on them, I just feel like shit."

"This anger is not you."

I sigh. "It's just so much easier with you. You always know what to say and what not to say."

He squeezes my hand. "And how's the knee feeling? We'll have to ice it when we get back."

"Ugh. This stupid knee has set me back in every way. I am really getting frustrated!"

"You can't rush an ACL injury. Keep going the way you are, and you'll be up and running in a few more months."

"Yeah, I know."

"You know the sexiest thing about you? You're so damn mentally strong. You take any challenge and get through it. You flip a switch in your brain and can left foot, right foot your way through anything."

"Yeah, and on the flip side, I have PTSD to deal with."

"But you get through it."

"It's crippling me."

"Well," he grins. "Your determination is a big turn-on."

"So being headstrong is one positive the military taught me!"

He wraps his arms around me. "So...think we can find you something less physical to do to keep yourself busy?"

"Actually, I've been thinking of going back to school."

"Oh yeah?"

"Yeah. For paramedic training. I took a bunch of medic courses in the Army. I really liked them, and I like helping people."

"That's a great idea. Especially if you plan to keep hurting yourself all the time!"

GOOD PLAN

Oh, Kelsi.

What a great idea.

Go back to school!

The type of environment you've never been able to thrive in, studying things that will trigger you constantly, all so that you end up with a career you will never be able to stomach.

I have lots of paramedics.

With you, I will get a paramedic and a vet in one.

Thanks!

TWENTY-ONE

The Beginning

2014

After a quick shoulder check, I merge into the right lane. A dirty older-model white sedan blares its horn. "Sorry! Shit!" I've cut him off.

I continue driving onto the bridge that will take me home, and that same white car speeds around me, forcing me onto the shoulder.

"What the actual hell?"

After pulling over to the side of the road, there's a banging on my windshield, and when I look up, a South Asian man screams, "Roll down the window!"

My heart rate speeds up. I reach to my left and make sure my doors are locked. I squeeze my eyes shut to avoid looking at him and use my right hand to feel through my purse for my phone and my switchblade. I hope to need only one of these tools today.

He continues to bang on my windshield, and I yell back, "Get the *fuck* away from my car."

I dial 911. "What is your emergency?"

I speak loudly into the phone. "I am being assaulted by a man on the Alex Fraser Bridge, and you better send someone quickly."

The man sees that I'm calling the police and rushes back to his car before speeding away.

The operator asks me for the license plate number, and I give it to her.

After we hang up, I realize my hands are gripping the steering wheel so tightly that my fingers are cramped. I release the wheel and call Brady.

"Hey, what's up?"

"So, I just cut off a car on the bridge, and a guy banged on my windshield—"

"Shit, Kels. Are you okay?"

"Yeah, I'm okay, but I wanted to tell you that he looked South Asian, and I didn't totally lose it. I might be getting better!"

As soon as I walk in the door, I drop my keys and my purse, then head straight for our bedroom. I change into shorts and sneakers, grab a bottle of water, lock the door, and start to run.

I can't believe the nerve of that guy. With every breath of fresh air, a bit of tension leaves my shoulders. As my muscles warm up, I quicken my pace until I find my stride. What was he thinking, banging on my car like that? I reach the path to the beach, and my knees welcome the switch from pavement to gravel. Finally, my sneakers hit the boardwalk.

I run till I no longer see the enemy in the face of the driver of that white car. But I dread going to sleep tonight, because I already know what nightmare I'll be served.

RUN

Run as much as you want to.
Let yourself believe it's helping.
As if you could run away from me.
From those images that repeat in your head.
From the smells and the sounds.

You can't outrun me, you stupid girl.

But sure, go ahead and try.

I'll catch up with you in your dreams.

Socially, school has never been easy for me. I can't relate to my peers any easier now than I could in high school, so I am proud of finishing the course. It will take months of additional training, however, if I want to be a paramedic, and I just don't have it in me.

I'm curled up on the couch with Tuck, a cup of tea, and a book, trying to convince myself that I'm not a failure.

"Hey, babe," Brady calls when he gets home from work.

"Hey, Roo!"

Tuck jumps off the couch, arches his back, and has a good stretch before running over to Brady. He comes into the living room carrying the cat. "You look cozy."

"I am." He reaches down to kiss me with a curious slowness. "How was your day?"

"Good!" He starts unbuttoning his shirt. "I'll go get changed if you're ready to go?"

"Go?"

"For our usual run. To the beach."

"Tonight?"

"Yeah, why not?"

"It looks like it might rain." Tuck joins me on the couch again, pushing his nose into my hand for a head rub.

"So?"

"Okay, if you insist, but you are ruining Tuck's evening plans."

"Tuck will get over it."

It's a cool evening, but the scenery makes it worthwhile as we run down the path to the ocean. The dark sky is threatening rain, and a bank of fog is moving in so that we can barely see past the pier.

"I just love it here," I say, gravel crunching beneath my sneakers.
"Me too."

"Your pace is slower than usual. You okay, Roo?"

"Yeah. I'm just a bit tired."

"You're the one who wanted to come out tonight, weirdo!"

After a little while, we get to the bottom of the hill and cross to
the beach, where a bunch of weathered old logs have washed in from
the ocean. "Let's sit down and take a break," he says.

"Sure." We sit on one of the dryer logs, watching the fog
drifting into shore. It looks almost dreamy with a faint glow from
the pier lights.

I check to see why Brady isn't sitting with me, and he is down on
one knee. "Brady Sheren, what are you doing?"

A huge smile lights up his entire face. "Will you marry me?"

I knew the minute I met him that I wanted to be with him forever,
so I don't hesitate when I answer. "Yes!" I squeal as he puts a dazzling
diamond ring on my finger.

Tears stream down my face, and I am happier than I have
ever been.

I feel happy.

I FEEL!

It's one of those rare moments when I truly feel like I'm taking
part in my own life. Everything seems real: the ring, his smile, the
tears on my cheeks. There is no shadow, no tap on my shoulder
saying: *remember.*

"I love you, Brady." I rest my forehead against his, feeling each
word. "I. Love. You." He wraps me in his arms and softly kisses me,
our breath and hearts locking forever. I love him, and he loves me,
and this is all that matters in the world. Not a thing or a person can
ever take this away from me. Maybe this is what each day will now
feel like when my battle is finally over.

CRASHING THE PARTY

Remember, I'm your main man.

I'll take you down the aisle to Hell again and again, render you helpless at the tiniest trigger.

Make you look foolish in front of a crowd.

I will hold on to you, no matter who comes into your life.

Love holds nothing to my power.

"Congratulations!" Dr. Passey says after I finish sharing my proposal story and showing off my beautiful engagement ring. "You look happy."

"I actually *feel* happy." I smile authentically as I sink back farther in my chair.

"The talk therapy has been going well. But we still need to find something new for you to focus on. I think you should try art therapy."

I chuckle. But the doctor isn't laughing.

"You're serious? Do we really think I'm the art therapy type? Sitting home making paper snowflakes isn't for me."

"Mindfulness is one of the best ways to deal with flashbacks and triggers. If we can absorb you in something in the here and now, focusing with your hands, PTSD won't have any power over you."

"I'm not making any promises, but I'll give it a try."

On my way home, I think about different forms of art I might actually be interested in. I decide to try a Michaels craft store for some inspiration, and the choices are overwhelming. I wander down the aisles from painting to knitting, from pottery to sewing, stopping when I reach the jewelry-making section. I run my hands over some beads, elastic, and wires, thinking it may be good to keep my brain and my hands busy making something. I buy some little pliers, wire, and string. I don't want any of the cheap plastic beads, but I know of a shop not far from here that sells natural stones and crystals.

With nothing but time on my hands, I pop in on the way home and talk to the salesperson.

The shop smells like incense, and salt lamps provide a calming glow. "I've heard different types of stones and crystals can be healing."

"Very much." A smile crosses her long-boned face. "What type of properties are you looking for?"

"I don't even know where to start, but I guess whichever stones are the most grounding?"

"I'd recommend hematite. It's the ultimate grounding gemstone for the body." She places a silver-gray stone into my palm, her stacked bracelets clicking on her wrist. "When it touches your skin, it feels like you're being sucked down into the earth. And it also eliminates negative energy, drawing it from you into itself."

I grab a handful of the stones. Anything can help.

She holds out a black stone next. "This one always has my back. Onyx. It stomps out negative thought patterns that come from fear. It's a root chakra stone."

I close my hand around it.

"What are you planning on doing with these stones?"

"Making a bracelet, I think."

"Combine it with these black crystals." Her long, ring-laden fingers choose a few stones from a bowl. "Onyx offers protection and security, while selenite provides clarity and new beginnings."

By the time I've gathered a selection, and she shows me how to string them properly, I have a plan for tomorrow, and I'm actually excited. This idea of art therapy might not be so crazy after all.

ROCKS

Art therapy is the perfect thing for you to do.

You keep on pretending that you can get better.

And I'll be here to prove you wrong every single time.

I wake from a deep sleep, but not from a nightmare this time. The words, *her, her, her* repeat in my head over and over. I don't know what they mean, but I am paying attention. Anxious to get started on my bracelet, I hop out of bed before Brady does, put on jeans and a T-shirt, start a pot of coffee, and set my supplies out on the kitchen table.

I don't know what the hell I'm doing, but I'm doing something.

Brady comes into the kitchen, freshly showered and shaven, and kisses me. "Looks like you have plenty to do today."

"I'm excited to get started!"

He pours coffee into his travel mug and sets down a cup for me next to my beads. "I'm going to work, Roo. Have fun."

"You too!"

I pour a selection of beads into my palm then set them on the table. One by one I string them on the elastic. Each time I choose a bead, I'm thinking only about what I'm doing in the moment. No other thoughts occupy my mind, one bead at a time, until I've finally finished my first bracelet.

I push the finished product onto my wrist, hold out my arm to admire my work, and smile. Within this short time, I've created something. I snap a photo of it and text it to Dr. Passey: *Look, i'm art therapying.*

I close my hand around a selenite stone and hold it.

New beginnings.

I cut another string, line up a few other stones, and start to bead another bracelet.

The door creaks open. "Hey, Kels!"

"You're home already?"

"It's five," he calls from the hallway.

"No...it is?" I look at my watch, then back to the few loose stones on the table.

Brady's lips are on my forehead. "Wow, you've been busy. And look at that smile!"

The table is covered in bracelets, and the hours have dissolved. There's a serenity within that I haven't experienced since my Tae Kwon Do days. My gaze is cast on the jewelry in front of me rather than the thoughts that usually clamor in my mind. I have spent an entire day working, and for the first time in years, my brain isn't on fire.

FAILURE

You think it's that easy to be rid of me?

It's only a matter of time.

You'll fail at this like you've failed at everything else.

Should I make a list?

Team sports, Tae Kwon Do, math, college, Afghanistan, friendships…need I go on?

TWENTY-TWO

Finding Meaning

"How did he do it?" Sadness seeps into me as I slide down the wall. Tuck trots over to me and rubs his head against my foot. I stroke his back, warming my shaking hands in his soft tangle of fur. I'm so numb to the news of another vet's suicide that I can't even manage tears.

"Hung himself." Watson's voice breaks.

I think back to the noose that was hanging in front of our tent when we first got to FOB Ramrod. "Shit," is the only word I can manage, and then thoughts from Afghanistan flood my brain. I should be sad, but I am empty. Numb. My thoughts start to close in and then go nowhere, sitting heavy on my heart.

For a moment, I'm lost, staring back at the same wall, and then Tuck licks my hand, his sandpaper tongue pulling me back to this world of hope. I won't give in to this and linger here. I am stronger than that.

"How are you doing, Kels?" he asks.

"With my PTSD—I'm actually doing better than I have been in years." I take a deep breath to control my anger. "But hearing

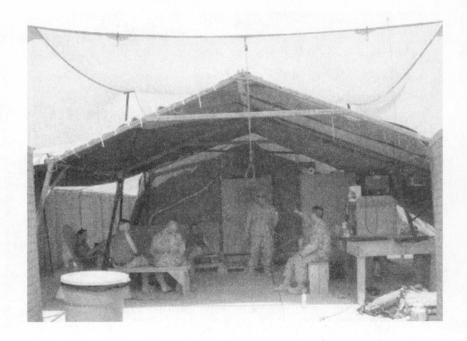

about another suicide pisses me off. When is someone going to do something?"

There's a pause on the line, and then Watson says, "Nobody's going to do anything, Burns. Nobody cares about us after we do the job we're sent to do."

"Well, *I* care. This has to stop. I've lost more friends to suicide than I lost while serving overseas."

"Aye. Me too. Hey, Burns?"

"Yeah?"

"A brilliant man will find a way to not fight a war."

"*Pearl Harbor*, 2001." When I hang up the phone, I turn back to my beading as a distraction, sliding each stone onto the string for someone I have lost to war. They have never left me. Never. And I have to do something to help veterans. It's an epidemic that nobody is doing anything about, or even talking about. Whether I can help or not, I'm going to try.

JOIN US

Another one of your comrades lost the war at home.

He's the lucky one.

His battle is over now.

You're the dummy who won't give in.

You're the dummy who keeps suffering—by choice.

Brady and I sit in the candlelit glow of the Cactus Club Cafe in White Rock for dinner with Rick and Shelley. I take a bite of my salad and wash it down with a sip of sangria.

Everyone at the table is silently chewing at the moment, so I take the opportunity to blurt out my news. "I'm going to start a jewelry company!"

Without any hesitation, Brady looks over at me and says, "Okay, I'm in. What do you need?"

Shelley laughs, her dark blonde hair reflecting the candlelight. "Where did this come from? Why jewelry?"

"I'm not sure why, but I just have to do this. I think I'm on to something with these bracelets I've been making. There might be a way to donate proceeds to support veterans who are falling through the cracks."

"That's just wonderful." Rick leans forward. "Do you know anything about starting a jewelry business?"

I take a drink to steel myself, but before I can answer, Brady says, "You know what would be cool, Roo? If you used a spent casing in the bracelets."

"That is an amazing idea."

"Do you have any?"

"Casings? Every shooting range in Canada and the U.S. has spent casings we could collect and recycle. They would just need to be cut and polished. That would look badass."

"I think you're on to something pretty special." Brady raises his glass. "Let's toast Kelsi." We clink. The sound echoes through the room as if lighting a new idea, and their smiles extend toward me, my body feeling supercharged and my heart excited. This smile on my face is real. I've never been happier than I am in this moment. Maybe there is something to those crystals and stones after all.

After we get home and change into our pajamas, I curl up next to Brady on the couch. He puts his arm around me. "You really do have a great idea. If you want, I'll help you build a website, and we can work on your brand. You've seen the kind of stuff I've done for my business."

I turn my head and look up at him. "Do you really think it's good enough? Do you think people will pay money for my bracelets?"

"I know they will." His sharp eyes are shining. "It's brilliant. You have the story and the idea, and I can help make it a business. Do you have a name in mind?"

"I think I want to call it Her Wearables." I move in closer to him, and no matter how hard I try, I can't get the silly grin off my face.

* * *

Two weeks later, I'm at the kitchen table with a pile of beads and brass bullet casings spread out in front of me, putting together one of my newly designed Warrior bracelets. Every time I look at one, I feel stronger in my resolve to keep going because of how far I've come.

I finish tying one of them when there's a knock at the door. "Hi, Rick! Brady's not here right now, but come on in."

"Actually, it's you I want to see." He enters the kitchen and takes a seat at my workbench/dinner table, the light shining off of his balding head.

"What's up? Want a coffee or tea or anything?"

"No, I'm fine." He doesn't look at me as he says this. He's distracted by my work area and the mess on the table.

I sit down beside him and start to tidy up.

He peers up at me over his glasses. "Kelsi, I think you have a really good idea here."

"Thanks, Rick."

"Brady told me about the Warrior bracelet, and I want to be the first person to buy one."

"Don't be silly. After everything you've done for me, I'll give you one."

"No, I will pay for it. You can't operate a business by giving your product away."

"Well, thank you! If you insist on paying for it, I'll take your money but will donate it to a veteran's charity."

"It's a deal. Tell me, where did the name come from?" Rick asks when I give him his bracelet.

"Well, I wanted a name that was connected to the military, and 'warrior' is a word that kept coming up. The casing on the bracelet is representative of being a warrior in your own life, no matter what your situation, and staying strong for your everyday life."

"I know you're going to be successful, Kelsi. Shelley and I are so proud of you." When he passes me a couple of twenty-dollar bills, I take them in my hand and give him a big hug. "Thank you! I have friends who want some, but you're my first official sale."

While Brady works on the website and brand for Her Wearables, I start looking online for women's stores in Vancouver that might carry the jewelry. One by one, I call the shops and ask for meetings, trying to get my foot in the door. It's hard, but I don't give up; this is where Army training serves me well.

For weeks I keep calling, one store at a time, until finally a woman on the other end of the phone doesn't shut me right down. Instead, she sounds interested. "Sure, can you bring in your samples and a line sheet?"

"Of course I can," I answer confidently, although I have no idea what a line sheet is. "When's good for you?"

"Tomorrow?"

"Great! See you then."

I have a lot to learn, but I catch on quick, and I'm driven to make this work.

The next day, I visit the store with my samples and line sheet, which, I learned, is basically a list of prices, and play it cool while the manager looks at my bracelets, trying some on.

I admire some of the sparkly jewelry and accessory displays, watching her out of the corner of my eye the entire time.

"Your Warrior bracelets are so edgy. They're fantastic."

"Thank you!" My stomach is in knots while I wait for her to make a decision.

"Can we try a few styles and see where it goes?"

"Sure." I try my best to play it cool while suppressing the joy inside me. "That works for me."

"I just love the shell casings."

Suddenly, the metallic smell of hot brass fills my nose. As she runs her hands along the spent casing, my happiness fades and my brain locks. I stop listening. Her mouth moves, but in my mind, I am in Afghanistan, racing in to the grape hut and then holding onto Mick's boot.

My brow furrows and my jaw is set, and there's nothing I can do to bring my smile back. I'm still with the British, taking heavy fire as we try to get Mick's body parts out of there. The shop manager can see that she's lost me, and I want to sink into the ground and disappear. I'm a shell of the person I was just a few minutes ago.

I find the strength to leave some bracelets with her and finish the paperwork, but the moment I step out of the store, the same weight settles inside me. No matter how fast I walk, no matter how bright the sun, how promising the day, it doesn't shift. I have just enough strength to reach my car. My head presses against the steering wheel, and I blink away the tears until they push through and I collapse. "I can't keep living like this," I sob. "I can't do this anymore."

What are you supposed to do when you don't want to die, but you also don't want to live?

DON'T FORGET ME

You got a little arrogant there again, didn't you?

I think you forgot who was calling the shots for a minute.

Go ahead and pretend you're okay, if that's how you want to play this.

We both know the truth.

You can't take much more, can you?

TWENTY-THREE

Stress, Stress, Stress

January 2014

"You have a lot on your plate, Kelsi," Dr. Passey cautions, leaning back in his chair. "Planning a big wedding, making jewelry, and running a business? Stress will make your symptoms worse, so be aware of that. How are you managing?"

"I'm doing okay."

He raises an eyebrow. "It would be understandable if you were struggling with things right now."

After all these years working with Dr. Passey, he knows I'm not being honest with him. I take a deep breath. "I'm not doing okay." As the words leave my mouth, I feel a wave of relief and clutch at my sweater as tears flow.

He pushes a tissue box closer to me, and I grab one. "I can't shut the video reel off. It's like I try to do something good, and my brain attacks me with reminders of the Op over and over. I can't live like this. It's like a horror movie in my head. I know I chose to join the Army and to deploy, but I had no idea how much it would mess me up."

"Most people don't realize what it's like overseas for military personnel." He hands me another tissue. "But you're working your way through this, and you're going to be okay."

"I just wish I could shut it off. Planning the wedding is fun, and I'm actually selling my jewelry from the website Brady built, and at the store here locally that's carrying it. Life is good, but now that I feel things, I feel too much. I can't tell you which is worse, me feeling nothing at all to now being out there in the world, happy and working, and then slipping into pain and becoming completely hollow. It's scary because I don't know who I am."

"It's a process, Kelsi. We just have to work a bit more on managing your stress."

"I was a mess when I had nothing to do, and now I'm a mess with too much to do. I can't win."

The frustration doesn't leave me for the rest of the day, and while Dr. Passey's words are reassuring, it feels like it's been too long and too much of a struggle. Every moment at home is coated in anger, even as I scrub away at the grease-splattered backsplash and then scrape each plate off before loading it into the dishwasher.

"I said I'd do those," Brady calls from the couch.

"Yeah, I know you did," I mutter, "and you didn't do them."

"I was going to, but I wanted to sit down for a minute first."

I snatch our glasses and utensils from the counter with such a speed that they clang against one another.

"And I need them to be done now, so I'm doing them." I'm angry at the dishes, the store clerk, car drivers, heck, I'm even angry that Tuck is at my feet. Most importantly, I'm angry at myself, this boggled brain of mine. "It's not a big deal, Brady."

"Sorry, Roo."

I noisily finish stacking everything and switch the dishwasher on before joining Brady on the couch.

"Kels, is everything okay?"

I lower my head. I want to apologize, but I can't. Not yet. I hate that I keep blowing up at him over nothing.

"Hey..." He rubs my hand. "What's going on?"

When I put my head on his shoulder, he wraps his arm around me. "When you wanna talk, we can talk, okay?"

Tuck joins us on the couch, and we just sit there for a few minutes before I finally speak. Quietly, I say, "I didn't mean to snap at you. I'm sorry."

"It's okay."

"I think the stress of the wedding and everything has me really overwhelmed, and I'm getting triggered like I was in the beginning."

"Have you talked to the doctor about this?"

"Yeah."

"And?"

"It's always going to be important for me to reduce my stressors and recognize my triggers, and I'm trying, but it's a lot right now."

"We'll get through it."

"You still love me, right?"

"I still love you."

"You're never going to leave me?"

"I'm never going to leave you. We're like Lego pieces. We just fit together." Brady kisses me on the forehead, and I melt into him. Every rise and fall of his chest behind me is another reason for me to keep breathing.

LOVER

Know who else is never going to leave you?
Me.
And I'm going to ruin your marriage.
Watch me.

In the months that follow, Brady and I have a beautiful wedding with all of our favorite people there supporting us. I'm spending my days making jewelry, and I'm keeping up my weekly visits with Dr.

Passey and Dr. Mok. I also give Brady the surprise of his life when I tell him we're expecting a baby.

For our first ultrasound, Brady comes along, and we are so excited to get a peek at this little creature living in my belly. I'm ready to burst because my bladder is so full for the test, but it's not the first time in my life I've been uncomfortable, and I know it won't be the last.

Brady squeezes my hand, and the ultrasound technician rubs cold jelly on my stomach. She moves her instrument around, and I distract myself from having to pee by trying to make out the shape of a baby on the ultrasound screen.

"Is everything okay?" Brady notices the technician is having a hard time finding something.

"It's still quite early to see anything," she explains. "How about you come back next week when the baby is a bit larger?"

We leave without a photo, but the whole experience opens a new door—there is life inside of me. Nothing has changed since the day before, nothing that anyone can see. Brady and I walk through a crowded lobby passing a man in a turban, and I barely notice. We get stuck in a traffic jam with people honking their horns, and I just smile softly and hold his hand tighter. Everything I've gone through in my life was worth it, if that's what was required to bring me to this moment.

The following week, I go through the same routine and wait nervously for news that our baby is healthy. It doesn't matter really, whatever state our child is in—I am a mother, and I will do anything to protect that beating heart inside of me.

"Kelsi." A nurse stands with the door open to a long hallway. "The doctor would like to see you."

I take a seat in the little room and text Brady, *I think something's wrong*. In that silence, I ponder my entire life, everything I would go through again, five times over, if it means our baby is okay.

My doctor enters the room, places the file onto the desk, and folds her hands. "I'm so sorry to tell you this," her voice lowers, "but we can't find a heartbeat. I'm afraid you've lost the baby."

My shoulders fall, and I feel sick as I bring my hands to my stomach, wishing Brady was here. How will we tell our families that there won't be a baby? Everyone was so excited. This time it isn't my brain that shuts down. It's fully awake, taking in his words again and again, trying to make sense of it all. It's my heart that breaks, and I can't find my breath.

Fear grips me, more than any panic ever has. And before I know it, darkness spreads through my thoughts, clouding my mind. A montage takes me back to Afghanistan, to places I never wanted to revisit again. I look at my face in the mirror and close my eyes to what I see. I thought this was over for me, but now there is no hope of being saved. It's. My. Fault.

"What did I do wrong?"

"Nothing, these things happen," she says gently.

"Was it my medication?"

"No." His voice lightens. "The good news is that you were able to get pregnant. You're young and healthy, and it will happen again."

LOSS

This is just what we needed to help you feel weak again.

I'm back!!

"My nightmares are more vivid and horrible than they ever have been. They're even worse than the ones I had when I finished my op." I feel my eyes well up. "Ever since the miscarriage."

"It's been a stressful year for you since you lost the baby." Dr. Passey pushes a box of tissues toward me.

"I know, but I was becoming so hopeful for the future, and I really felt I was getting better." My foot taps nervously as I fidget with my bracelet. "I just want this to go away. Is that so much to ask?"

"PTSD has a funny way of lying dormant until you feel like you're moving forward, and then it reaches out and punches you in the face. You've come a very long way, Kelsi."

"But I feel like I stepped right back to where I started when the doctor gave me that news. It was like a dagger into my world."

"But remember the good thing?"

I shrug. "What's that?"

"You feel. You cry. You love. You wanted that so much, and it hasn't left you. It's just that all the good feelings are stronger, but all of the bad feelings or hard times are also now harder. With no emotion, you kind of operate at this middle baseline with very little variation, but that has changed for you."

"I'm really trying, but I have two moods; either nothing goes wrong and the world is lovely, or something triggers me and my brain goes dead."

"I think it's time to try medical marijuana, Kelsi. You're trying to get pregnant, and it will be safer for you to use during pregnancy than other pharmaceuticals. Many of my patients are having great success with it."

"Actually, I've been doing some research, and I think it might be time to give it a try. Screw the stigma."

BOO-HOO

You didn't actually think you could be a parent, did you?

What are your qualifications?

Weak.

Loser.

That's not going to cut it, is it?

I'm never going away.

Never. Are you prepared to live with me forever?

TWENTY-FOUR

The New People

June 2015

After cleaning up some brass casings from the front deck of our new home, which, I am aware, makes me look like a crazy person, I decide to take a walk down the street to where a moving truck has been parked all day and introduce myself to our new neighbor.

We just moved into this cul-de-sac, and I'm starting to recognize the people who live here now. It seems to be a tight-knit little community, and I love how everyone has kids and seems to be so friendly.

I push Gould's Oakleys up onto my head, knock on the door of my new neighbor's house, and a woman with dark brown hair answers. "Can I help you?"

She is about two inches taller than me, forcing me to look up to meet her gaze. "Hi! I'm Kelsi. My husband Brady and I live in that house over there." I smile as I point to our home.

"Oh, you're the one with veteran plates on your car?"

"Yep!"

"Well, my husband and children are Muslim. Does that mean you're going to kill them?"

Those words knock the wind out of me more than a kick in the stomach would. My smile folds into a grim line, and in my stunned state I manage to mutter, "I don't kill children." Almost robotically, my feet move away from the house, and I barely notice my neighbors Tina and Shelley as they pass me.

"Hi, Kelsi!"

I don't even look up.

"Hey, Kelsi?" Tina gently holds on to my arm. "What's wrong?"

I stop, try to relax my shoulders, unclench my teeth, and I explain what just happened.

Tina looks at me, agape. "Seriously?"

I nod.

Shelley adjusts the purse strap on her shoulder. "What an awful thing for her to say to you."

"Yeah, pretty terrible."

Tina shakes her head and lets out a deep sigh. "You know that's not what the majority of people think, right?"

"Whatever, I just need to cool down. I'm going to go home and bang on some bullet casings."

"Hey," Shelley says. "A few of us are meeting for drinks tonight. You should join us and see that not everyone in the cul-de-sac is awful."

Somewhat reluctantly, I go to the party, knowing I can't stare at another wall as a coping measure.

"Welcome, Kelsi!" I'm greeted by a smiling woman on the opposite side of the door.

"Thanks for the invite." I hand her a bottle of wine.

"Oh, thank you! I'll add this to the collection. Would you like a glass of red?"

"Yes, please."

I scan the space until I spot Tina and Shelley, and they wave me over from across the room.

"Kelsi, this is..." Shelley starts naming people, and as I try to remember the faces, I feel hot and overwhelmed. I take a deep breath and feel very thankful for the therapist-approved marijuana I smoked before coming over here.

"Everyone, this is Kelsi." Shelley picks up my wrist and shows off the bracelets I'm wearing. "Kelsi has started a fabulous company called Her Wearables. She's planning to donate money to programs for veterans and first responders with PTSD." She points to the crowd with her wide grin. "You all have to buy one."

"Did you bring any with you?" asks Tina. She's one of many RCMP officers who live in the "sac," and I really hope she can't smell the marijuana on me.

I nervously take a sip of wine, trying to contain my excitement. "No, but I can text Brady to bring some over if you want."

"Please do." She claps her hands.

"Okay!" I take out my phone and text Brady. *They want to buy some of my pieces. Can you please bring some over?*

"How did you get into making bracelets, anyway?" Tina reaches for my wrist to take a closer look.

"Well, my psychiatrist recommended that I try art therapy to help with my PTSD, and it really worked. It's crazy how relaxing it is to put beads on string."

"I love that idea." Tina's kind eyes hold my gaze for a moment. "If you ever need help with it, would you let me know? I could use some relaxation myself."

"Yeah, that would be great. Thanks!"

A voice comes from behind. "Your work is beautiful!"

"Thank you!" I say as I turn around. The woman admiring my bracelet has dark brown eyes and hair and an accent I can't quite place.

"My name is Asma." She extends her hand.

I take her hand. "Kelsi."

"Yes." She smiles. "I know! I'd love to see more of your pieces, but I have to go now—baby at home."

"Sure, come over anytime," I say. My heart breaks a little bit at the thought of the baby we lost.

"Oh, if you came to me, that would be great. That way, my child won't destroy your home."

I laugh. I can already tell I'm going to like this woman.

"I can do that."

"Can I put my number in your phone?"

"Yeah, here you go." I pass my phone over to her, and she adds herself to my contacts.

"I'll be home all day tomorrow."

"Sounds good."

ACCENT

```
You're chatting with the enemy.

Can't you picture her in a burka?

If she wore a headscarf, would you have spoken
to her?

Are you really letting down your guard?

Perhaps you need a reminder.
```

"Thanks so much for coming!" Asma says when I knock on her door. "You picked a great time to visit, because it's nap time!"

"Oh, you're welcome."

"Can I get you a coffee or tea, juice?"

"I'm fine for now, but thanks."

"All right, come on in, let's sit in the living room."

Asma leads me to a big leather couch, and we both sink into it.

"So, how do you like the neighborhood?" she asks while I pass her some pieces of jewelry.

"We really like it."

"It's a great place to raise a family."

"Seems that way. Brady and I are trying for a baby."

"Oh, that's great! Trying is the best part."

We both laugh. Then she asks, "Are you from BC?"

"No, actually, I grew up in a small town in Ontario."

"Oh, you're from out east. It must be hard being away from your family." She tries on a bracelet and touches the stones. "I'd love to buy this one, please."

"Sure! Thank you. And yes, it is tough being away, but we talk every day. Where are you from?"

"I'm from Serbia."

"That is much farther away!"

She smiles warmly. "I heard what happened to you with the new family that moved down the street. Listen," she continues, "I'm Muslim, and I don't feel that way about you, if it makes you feel any better."

My breath catches in my throat. I look at this tall, thin, fair-skinned woman. I never would have expected that she's Muslim. Every instinct I have says to leave, but I reprimand myself. *Kelsi, you're not in Afghanistan anymore. This woman is not the enemy.*

I feel myself shutting down, and suddenly the marijuana in my purse is screaming at me to take it outside. I can't find it in me to speak. My face is flushed, and I start to break into a sweat. I have to respond to her. "Thank you for saying that."

"I understand war. It wasn't fair of her to say such things to you. Do you mind if I ask, how has your transition to civilian life been?"

Looking into Asma's dark brown eyes, I don't see the hatred that looked at me through the burkas in the compounds I searched. Rather than coldness, I sense warmth, compassion, and curiosity. "It's actually been really, really hard. I was medically discharged with PTSD, and I never got any support from the military."

"PTSD is a real crisis. I hope you're getting some sort of help."

"I don't tell many people this, but the biggest lifesaver for me has been cannabis."

"Hey, girl, whatever works!" Asma curls her feet up underneath her. "I'm not here to judge."

I'm so relieved by her reaction that I feel safe asking her something that's been burning on my mind. "I have a weird question for you."

"Sure, what is it?"

I turn toward her, nervously twisting my Warrior bracelet. "Will you teach me about the Qur'an?"

She seems a bit surprised but answers right away. "Of course. May I ask why?"

"I want to understand Islam better."

A wide smile spreads over her face. "Well. The absolute first thing you need to know is that the Taliban's extremist version of Islam is not practiced outside of Afghanistan."

She talks about Allah and prophets and messengers. I'm glued to her every word until a cry comes from the baby monitor. "Be right back," Asma says as she rushes off to the nursery.

I hear her soothing voice through the monitor, and as she softly coos to the baby, all I dream about is holding a child of my own. The cries fade, and as I listen to Asma sing to the child, I feel my eyes start to well up. In a minute she's back, sitting on the couch next to me.

"Sorry about that," she says. "Where were we?"

I twist again to face her. "You were telling me about Jesus being mentioned in the Qur'an. It sounds so similar to what I grew up hearing in Catholic school."

"I think all religions are about peace and love at the root of things."

I shift my position and hug an oversized throw pillow. "It's so ironic that religion is also at the root of most wars."

RELIGION

There's one war that religion has nothing to do with—the one you're waging now.

Against me.

And this is the type of battle that doesn't end until everyone is dead.

"Look at you two, still on top of each other all the time," my mother-in-law teases.

Brady and I are snuggled on their couch by the Christmas tree during the yearly gift exchange.

"Here, Papa." Brady passes a gift to his eighty-nine-year-old grandfather. "This one is for you from Kelsi and me."

His face brightens with a big smile. "You know you don't have to be getting me presents. You should be saving your money!"

"Open it!" My stomach is full of butterflies, watching him carefully pull off the paper.

"Hmm...what could it be?"

Shelley, Rick, and Nessy all watch in anticipation. We haven't told any of them what we got for Papa this year.

He opens up the box and pushes aside the light pink and blue tissue paper. He reaches into the bottom of the box and pulls out the sonogram photo, bringing it to his face to study it closer. "Oh, you're having a baby!"

"Yes! And Papa, if it's a boy, we're naming him Jack, after you."

"Well. I can't think of a nicer gift than that! Congratulations!"

"Oh!" Shelley squeals. "We've been waiting for this announcement since last year!" She comes over and gives me a tight squeeze while Rick shakes Brady's hand.

"How far along are you?" Nessy throws her tattooed arms around my neck.

"Just a couple of months."

"How are you feeling?" Shelley asks.

"I'm feeling really good. My treatment is going well, and I love being pregnant."

"Well, you're glowing," she says.

Both Brady and I wear a permanent grin for days after sharing the news, and months later, our perfect little Jack-a-Roo enters the world ahead of schedule. As promised, we name him Jack.

BABY BLUES

Let it all out, Kelsi.

You have something new to live for now.

But that isn't making things any easier, is it?

I'm counting on it.

A month after having Jack, I'm sitting beside him and a basket of laundry, crying. I slept through Tina's visit earlier when she dropped off some meals for us, and I'm so upset that I missed her. Brady is working, but his mom's here to help me. She rubs my back while I sob. "It's okay, Kelsi. Let it out."

"I can't stop crying." I blow my nose with a damp wad of tissues. "I'm so tired. I'm the worst mother ever," I manage between sobs.

"It's normal to be emotional after you have a baby, but how about we make an appointment for you to see your doctor, just in case? They did say that postpartum depression (PPD) would probably happen for you, so you should talk to someone."

PPD + PTSD

I know PPD!

We go way back.

It's fun when we both get invited to the party!

Before my six-week checkup, I stop at the grocery store to pick up diapers and a few other items. I put Jack's car seat carrier in the shopping cart and head for the baby aisle.

The store is crowded, and shoppers are rushing past me. I scan ahead of the cart, looking for anything out of place. *There are no IEDs here, Kelsi. You're okay.*

Beads of sweat trickle down my back. Taking a breath, I steer us to the diapers and face a wall of options that all look identical. "Which brand have we been using?" My eyes dart at the different sizes and prices. I grab a package of them, and suddenly I can't remember which size we need. Setting the packages down, I reach into my bag to see what diaper size I have in there, to compare.

Jack whimpers from the car seat, so I stand up and lean over the cart. "Hi, Jack-a-Roo, we're almost done!" He starts to fuss, and my face turns red. "I can't remember which diapers we need, bubby."

Tears fill my eyes, and I break down crying in the diaper aisle. Frantically, I reach out for my phone. *Brady, please pick up diapers.*

Abandoning my cart, I pick up the carrier and the diaper bag to take Jack and me to our appointment.

GOOD

Things are playing out exactly how I planned.

When PPD and I work together, we get the job done much faster.

I search a compound filled with women in burkas, each of them holding a baby. "Stand by the wall and put your babies on the floor in front of you," I yell coldly.

I can't see any of the women's eyes through the screens of their burkas. They look like shadows. All of the babies cry. I start searching the first woman, patting her down. The woman next to her reaches out and grabs my weapon while the others hold me and tie my hands behind my back. I am outnumbered. The babies cry and cry, and the woman points the gun at me and pushes the barrel into my cheek.

SAY UNCLE

Listen to the baby crying.

He's just like the ones you searched in Afghanistan.

Can you hear them?

How many of your mortar rounds landed on babies?

And their mothers?

That's the thought I want you to go to bed with tonight.

You're a monster.

Just like that neighbor of yours thinks you are.

You don't deserve to live.

"Roo, wake up. It's okay." Brady's voice whispers in my ear.

"The babies are all crying," I mumble.

"It's only Jack. Are you okay? I'll get up with him."

My face is soaked with tears. "I'm okay. I think I'll get up with him."

"Are you sure?"

"Uh-huh."

I put on my slippers and go next door to Jack's nursery. "Hey, bubby, what's wrong?" I ask quietly. His little cry is so sad, but it feels good to be needed. After a quick diaper change, I scoop up his tiny warm body and sit on the rocking chair with him. He knows what he wants, and I bring him to my breast for a feeding. As I watch him wrap his pink hand around my thumb, I can't help but cry. But I cry at everything since he's been born.

"I like being your mom, Jack," I whisper to him, sniffling through my tears. "I'm crying because I'm happy. I think. Or maybe because I'm exhausted."

I run my finger over his perfect little pink forehead.

"I never imagined loving someone as much as I love you, Jack." My finger looks so huge in his wrinkled hand.

"Hey, guess what? I'm almost ready to donate my first check to Honour House, that place for vets and their families to go and get better when they're sick like Mommy."

We rock together for a few minutes until he's milk-drunk.

"The jewelry we're making is going to actually help people. I hope that makes you proud one day."

Rocking and crying, I look at him for hours. PTSD is a fickle bastard; he likes to come out right when you feel like you've got a handle on your life and make it so you don't want to go to sleep—that's where the nightmares live.

My eyes start to grow heavier and heavier, so I set Jack back in his crib. I give him a kiss on his fuzzy warm little forehead and go back to bed, amazed at how good it feels to fill a baby's needs and proud that I've come far enough to keep myself and another human alive.

TWENTY-FIVE

A New Chapter

September 2015

"UGGHH!" I throw down my pliers.

"What's wrong with you?" Tina asks from her side of the basement workbench. The business has been relocated down here to accommodate our growth and the fact that it's annoying to work from the kitchen table. Tina has been working with me sometimes to help with her own workplace stresses. She's the closest thing I've had to a friend in...ever.

"I've been fighting with this stupid thing for twenty minutes."

"What did I tell you, Kels? No crying over tangled elastic. It's time for a break."

"Okay," I set down the pliers. "I have to call my parents back anyway."

"First, tell me what's bothering you?"

She's a pain in my ass in the best possible way.

"Since business has kind of exploded, I'm starting to drown."

"Remember, Kels, any time you're in a stressful situation, things are going to be harder for you. Are you sure this is what you want to be doing?"

"Yes." I take a sip of tea. "All this work is going to help veterans. But as things get busier with the business and with Jack, I'm getting triggered more. I feel like such a shit mom."

"How many times do we need to go over this, Kelsi? You're a good mother. This is PTSD talking. Don't let it make you think that."

"How can you say I'm a good mother when I'm on your doorstep every other day freaking out about something?"

"Because good mothers get help when they need it."

"Ugh, you're so annoying."

Tina laughs. "I know. As much as I don't agree with it—the cannabis is helping?"

"It's helping more than anything."

"Well, that's good, I guess. I still don't approve of it."

"I know you love me regardless."

My computer buzzes. "Oh, hang on a sec, Tina, Mom's calling on FaceTime."

"I have to go anyway." Tina gets up and gives me a quick hug as I answer the call.

"Hey, Mom!"

"Kelsi, you'll never guess what just happened." She has the biggest smile on her face.

"What? Why do you look so happy?"

"You know I'm driving for Kevin Hart's tour right now?"

"Uh-huh, yes."

"You need to come to the show in Vancouver, because he wants to meet with you!"

"Um, Kevin Hart does?"

"Yes! I've told him all about what you're doing, and he wants to meet you!"

"Oh my God, Mom, really?"

"Yes, really."

"Thank you!"

"I gotta go, sweetie, but I'll see you there."

* * *

Backstage at the Rogers Arena in Vancouver, I'm full of nerves as Kevin Hart's tour manager introduces us.

"We really enjoyed the show." My voice quivers, but Brady shakes his hand like they're old friends.

"Well, thank you for coming out. Your mother tells me that I need to meet you and see this jewelry you're making."

Hoping he can't tell how sweaty my palms are, I pass him a box of bracelets that I've made for him and his team. "These are for you."

"Thank you." He starts to look at them, studying them closely. I can't believe Kevin frickin' Hart is trying on my bracelets.

"Hey, these are great." He turns to Mom with a wide, toothy smile. "You were right, Cathy!"

I let out a quiet sigh of relief. "I'm glad you like them."

"Kelsi," he turns all his attention to me, "tell me about your company and where you want it to go."

"Well, I served in Afghanistan and was medically discharged with a diagnosis of PTSD. I tried a bunch of things over the years to help me get better, but making jewelry was the first one that really worked. Brady had the idea to use spent casings in the design, we patented the Warrior bracelet, and the rest is history."

"Very cool," he says.

My shoulders start to relax. "I want to donate profits to veteran programs to do something about the suicide crisis facing vets right now." I look him straight in the eye. "I want my friends to stop killing themselves."

We chat for a few more minutes until it's time for him to go. "Can we grab a photo?" Brady asks.

"Of course! Tag me, and I'll share it."

I'm practically vibrating with excitement. "Oh my God, thank you!"

"I have one word of advice, though," he offers with intense focus as he puts on a bracelet. "Change the name from Her Wearables.

Make it unisex, because if you want men to wear them too, you should think about that. Anyone can wear these."

We walk away from that meeting completely amped up about our business.

That night, Kevin Hart retweets our photo of him with his bracelet to his twenty-four million followers. In his tweet, he tells his followers why they should support us and how my company is helping vets.

"I have an idea for a new name," Brady mentions as we watch Twitter blow up after Kevin's tweet. "He's right, it has to be something gender-neutral."

"Whaddaya got?" I ask.

"I like the word 'brass,' because it's really military-sounding, but we can't really do anything with that for a trademark."

"It sounds cool, though!"

"Yeah, right? I did some brainstorming, and I kind of like the sound of Brass and Unity. It combines military and bringing people together, which is what you're doing."

"Brass and Unity," I repeat. "I love it!"

POPULARITY

Oh, Kelsi, what a wonderful favor you've done for me!

A celebrity has shared your business.

Now you have to pretend that you are an actual entrepreneur!

And you know that's going to come with a lot of stress.

Stress that you can't handle.

Wait right here while I wrap my hands around your throat and remind you who's boss.

Pacing the kitchen floor, waiting for Brady to get home from work, I bounce Jack on my hip. Finally, I hear him come in and rush over to give him a kiss. "You're *never* going to guess what happened today."

"Hey!" He reaches out for Jack. "What happened today?"

"I got a phone call from one of Beth Behrs's people."

"Beth Behrs, the actress from *2 Broke Girls*?"

"Yes!"

"Cool! Something to do with Brass and Unity?"

"Yeah, so she has an equine therapy program for sexual assault survivors and wants to work with us to raise funds."

"That's awesome, Roo!"

"But it gets better." I take a breath before I blurt, "She's going on Ellen's Twelve Days of Christmas Giveaways and wants to bring our jewelry on the show."

"Babe! That's insane!"

"I know! We're going to help so many people."

Still balancing Jack, Brady gives me a huge hug, and when he pulls away, he wipes a tear from my eye. "Do you feel happy, Roo?"

The smile on my face says it all.

* * *

It's now 2019, and I'm in my dressing room, getting ready to step onto the stage of *The Doctors*. Fixing my dark brown hair (I long ago said goodbye to the blonde of my childhood) I take a deep breath. I smooth my hands over my long dress and think about what I'll say. I can't believe I am in Los Angeles and about to appear on live television.

Beyond this door there are bright lights, and questions, and a live studio audience. But I am strong. I'm reminded of that every time I look at the bracelet on my wrist—I'm winning.

My phone vibrates from the coffee table, and I pick up. I smile when Watson's face flashes across the screen:

Knock 'em dead, Kelsi.

Thanks, bud.

Let me know when it airs.

Will do. Hey, Watty?

Yeah?

Thank you for always being there for me.

Ditto, Burns.

In my reflection, as I apply my lip gloss, I still see the girl who was bullied on the playground and betrayed by someone she trusted, and I see the young woman who fought bravely on the front lines in Afghanistan. But I also see a wife, a mother, a friend, a daughter, a sister, a lover, and a businesswoman. I see a veteran who is doing something to make the world a better place, which is all I ever wanted to do.

I don't see a broken soldier. I see a warrior. I see a survivor.

WRONG

    You will always belong to me—

No, I don't belong to you, PTSD. You belong to me. Fuck you.

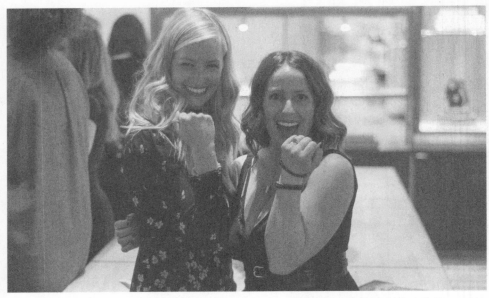

Top:
With Beth Behrs

Right:
With Kat Dennings
and Beth Behrs

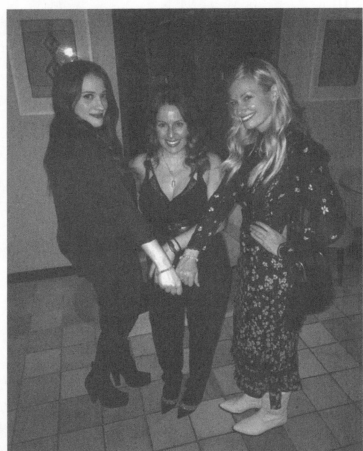

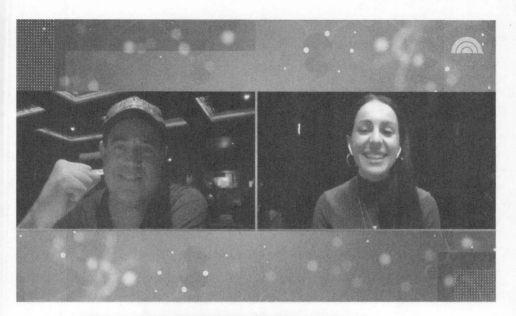

Top:
With Carson Daly

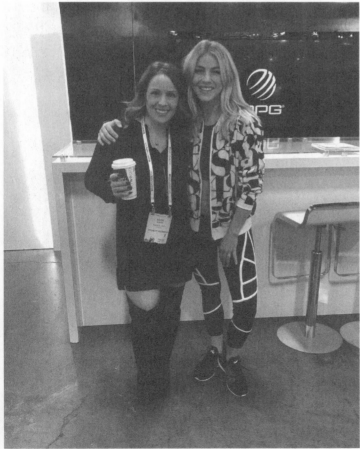

Left:
With Julianne Hough

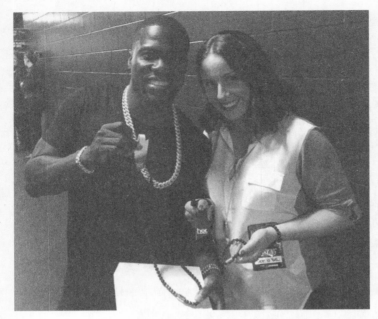

With Kevin Hart

*With Neal
McDonough*

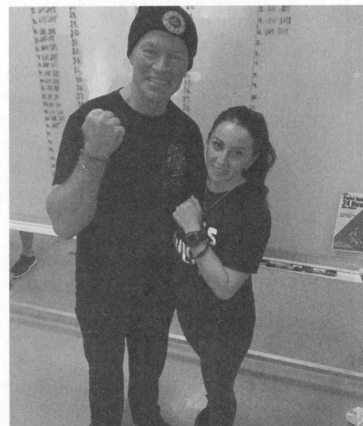

TWENTY-SIX

Healing

October 2020

In 2020, I started to do things a bit differently. We decided to start a podcast called "The Brass & Unity Podcast." My goal was to be able to have conversations with people who had wild life stories of heroism, triumph, struggle, and recovery that others could learn from. Come at it from a mental health lens, but with a twist and give listeners a chance to resonate with the guest. The goal was to be able to get others to give me completely different interviews than they had given other shows. To date, I believe I have been able to do that, and I plan to keep doing it for the rest of my life.

I wanted something different from what was already out there in the podcast world. Vulnerability, real raw vulnerability in all ways. I set out to do this in October 2020, and one of the first sponsors who came on board was called "Combat Flip Flops." One of the owners of this company is named Matthew Griffin, he was a U.S. Army Ranger, went to West Point, and worked on combat missions abroad. Brady and I had seen this amazing company on the entrepreneurial reality television show called *Shark Tank* a while back, and it was founded by two Army Rangers.

Brady suggested I reach out to them in an email, thinking they might be a good fit considering both brands and companies were working to make the world a better place. Within a few days, I got an email back.

"Hey, Kelsi! Casings in sunglasses, and casings in our flip-flops, we go together like peanut butter and jelly."

I was thrilled when I got this message; at this point, I hadn't thought I'd get a response, little alone so quick. Great customer service over there! I knew if I wanted to have this podcast take off, I would need top tier guests—serious hitters in their perspective spaces. Whether it was science, health, military, business, or otherwise.

So I took another risk and wrote back:

"Hey, Griff, would you like to be a guest on the show as well?"

To my surprise again, I got an email back the same day.

"Absolutely, Kelsi, when?"

"Next week?"

"Done."

WHOA! That's when the nerves kicked in; I got him booked, but now I needed to make sure I was ready for this interview.

That week, Griff was scheduled to be one of the first guests on the show. I had done some research on this guy, and he was solid as hell. Army Ranger, West Point grad. I knew what I had to do: Breathe and act like I've done this my whole life. Key word: act.

My mother and a few teachers (not all, ha ha) used to say, "let her talk, she will use her voice for something big one day."

The day of the interview came around, and I thought I was ready. Sure I was ready for the interview, but what came after was something I couldn't have made up even if I tried.

Griff leaned into the camera with a soft compassionate smile and was looking at me as if I had something on my face. He said "Kelsi, how ya doing?"

"I'm great, why do you ask?"

"Let's try that again," he says.

I was taken aback; I hadn't had someone ask me like that since Dr. Passey.

"Seriously, how are you doing?"

At that exact moment, it all came flooding forward, and I broke down; I cried and said, "I don't know, I'm trying so hard to move forward, but it's not getting any better. I'm doing everything I can and yet it's just not enough"

Griff leaned in and said, "Okay, well, have you ever heard of a medicine called ayahuasca?"

I replied "yes," but wasn't quite sure what it was or how it could help pull me from the slow decline that just never seemed to end.

He leaned in a little closer and said, "Let me tell you a little about ayahuasca and this organization called Heroic Hearts Project."

After our interview, Griff spent another hour of his time explaining to me what this plant-based medicine was and how it was helping not only him but so many veterans around him. He said he could connect me with the founder of Heroic Hearts Project and see if they could put me on a retreat.

I remember just saying "YES, PLEASE," over and over. I didn't wait a second, didn't speak to Brady about it, and just said yes.

It was this moment in time that I'll never forget. The fork in the road, the new path.

A week later, I was on a call with Jesse Gould, the founder of Heroic Hearts Project, going over what the medicine was, where it was, and how his project could help me. I didn't think I could get any better, I had come to the moment in my life where I figured, well this just is what it is. Little did I know, this, this was just the beginning of my true healing in a much deeper and profound way.

Just over a month later, I would be on a plane to a retreat with Heroic Hearts Project. I had little to no idea how much this experience would change my life, who I was, and who I would grow into. Once I landed, I was met with open arms by Griff and several of his special operations friends. These friends quickly became my pack, and people I could lean on for the rest of my life. They came from all walks of life, different cultures, and different upbringings. Different past careers in and out of the service, with one common denominator: We were all looking for relief in a deep way. A way that some just hadn't found yet, while some were further down the path.

We drove out to the location we would be at for the next three nights, where we would drink Ayahuasca in what are called ceremonies and learn things about ourselves in a very raw and vulnerable way. We would spend some time getting to know one another, why we were there, and what we were looking to get out of the ceremonies. At this time, I couldn't picture some of these guys being so open and vulnerable, but by the end of that weekend, I realized strong men don't hold their emotions in, they let them out and feel. That's true strength and courage.

The first night of ceremony was the most nerve racking. I had never felt anxiety like I had that night.

"Are you ready?"

"As ready as I will ever be, please just help the pain go away," I said.

We waited for night, the stars in the sky were so clear, clearer than I had ever seen. The deep blue and bright light of the moon, the crisp air and sounds of animals in the trees. Something felt different. There was a moment I felt as if everything in my life was now out of my hands, out of my control completely. My life, like the rest of those humans walking one in front of the other into the yurt, would change the second I stepped my foot across that doorway. Almost into another world, one I couldn't see or touch, yet one that was there sitting and waiting.

I walked slowly, cautiously over to my place in the yurt. I get comfortable on my four-inch bed with a blanket, and a bucket beside me in case I need to purge. I look over to my left, my right, and the guys across the yurt and smile, take a moment to thank my friend who introduced me to the medicine. This was my chance, my time to sit and give over control to something else. I had tried the prescribed medication—so many meds—the fitness, the food, the overall health, but I was not getting better.

The Mistro, as some call them, or shamans to others, took their place in the yurt and began blowing smoke all over themselves, cleansing and preparing the medicine.

I watched with such intensity, repeatedly saying over and over, "I'm open, I'm here, please help me heal this pain." My heart was heavy, it felt like someone was standing on my back holding me down, pulling me down to the depths. So much of my pain was inside, and it was becoming too heavy to carry any longer. The Mistros handed the container of Ayahuasca, after blowing smoke cleansing the container, to the assistant. We sat and waited as we were called one by one to the middle of the room where we would sit and be given a cup filled with this dark thick liquid.

I watched each person go one by one until it was my turn. I was so nervous at the thought of doing something wrong.

Had I made the right choice?

I couldn't back down now, so I took a moment and once again asked for help. I lifted the cup and poured back the entire amount and swallowed quickly. I stood up, said thank you, and made my way back. I saw everyone leaning up against the side walls, so I climbed onto my bed and did the same. My stomach began to turn, I was hot and then cold, hot again and felt weak. My anxiety was too much, and within twenty minutes I knew this wasn't going to stay in my stomach. I could feel it creeping up on my esophagus to the back of my throat and into my mouth. I quickly swallowed, and waited. Again it began to creep up once more, I swallowed again and I kept looking across the room, and another veteran saw this and had a little smirk. Again, I could feel it coming up, this time I couldn't hold it any longer,

"BLAAA," into the bucket the ayahuasca went. I was so embarrassed, I truly tried to keep it down, but my body couldn't bare it.

Yuck, the taste was just as bad going down as it was coming up!

We were all now ready, waiting to begin this journey.

The lights went down, and we sat in pitch black, waiting for the medicine to "open up."

"BREATHE."

"What?!"

"BREATHE." I heard the voice from somewhere keep repeating.

Oh, here we go. I was feeling something now. It's incredibly hard to describe in words, a feeling that only when felt could be understood. At first, I just kept hearing these words over and over—as if I wasn't breathing? I thought for sure I was breathing.

I looked down and thought, *Oh ya, I'm for sure breathing, right? Right??*

I was being told to take a deeper breath in and out, in and out. This instruction was coming from someone, somewhere, I couldn't place from where, but I felt my lungs expand as far as they could and then out like I was filling a hot air balloon. Over and over. The deeper the breath the further I began to fall into the medicine.

The colors and visuals were overwhelming as the healers sang their prayers, the patterns and spinning motions making my eyes roll back.

I was taken on a journey so deep that I feared for a second I couldn't come back. That I wouldn't; like I had finally done it. Like I had pushed myself over the edge. That edge that was in the back of my mind when I couldn't take the pain of living any longer. My body was still but my mind was gone, it was black. Absolute nothingness, the emptiness, the depths.

I felt something powerful take over my body; I began purging over and over. The assistant would come over and blow smoke in my face to relieve the pain I was feeling during the intense purging, allow me to catch my breath while I purged. I thrust my head in and out of my bucket, gasping for any air I could get. I had lost consciousness, and only right before I began to vomit once again would I come back into my body.

The experience was so intense, overwhelming really. The first three days sitting with the medicine was so deeply healing and profound. The affect it had on me was life-changing, soul-saving. Unlike any relief I had ever felt. I felt nothing and everything around me all at once, but it was the next hours and days ahead that would shape me in a way that allowed me to open up and accept a new way of healing.

Those next few days would be the transformation I needed to push on into a new point in my life. Physical pain was gone in areas of my body that had been previously broken. To this day, I'm still missing a decent amount of my collarbone from a mountain bike crash. Chronic pain in this area was causing me a ton of issues, and now it was just—gone. My soul was light, everything around me was light.

I felt a connection to everything around me, everyone around me. Anger was lifting, and I felt for the first time like life was possible now, in a really different way. If I did the work after ceremony and integrated this into my life.

I can do this.

Ayahuasca for me was a turning point that allowed a deeper healing that I was missing after years of traditional therapies. Don't get me wrong, there is a time and place for medications depending on needs. But for me, the standard meds weren't the answer.

Plant-based medicines had become a part of my life back in 2015 with the use of cannabis; it helped me get off all the pharmaceutical drugs that were hurting me more than helping me. The next step for me was realizing how much better I could feel if I looked for a non-traditional way of healing. Because I had such a forward-thinking doctor, someone who wasn't being paid off by the pharma companies and truly cared about his patients, I was being open to the world now in a different way, in the way people say, "Wow that's crazy timing?" or "How did you get into that situation?"

My answer to them is just this.

I was hurting so bad that I had no choice but to open myself up to the world in a vulnerable and deep way.

I was grateful to Griff, and am to this day, for introducing me to this medicine and those who provided it, Heroic Hearts Project, Jesse Gould, and their donors.

As I sit here writing this now, I am on a plane coming home from my ninth time sitting with the medicine. This time, Heroic Hearts Project gave me the blessing of traveling to Peru to sit with the medicine, in the birthplace of this true gift. I thought about this book a lot on this retreat, whether I would share the fantastical events that happen when sitting with the medicine, and I've come to the realization that I can be deeply vulnerable and still hold some of these stories for myself.

I have shared my stories publicly before on large podcasts and fully given myself over in the deepest most vulnerable ways in interviews with a lot of trust, to those I thought I could trust, only to have them blow up in my face.

Not this time. I hold the power now, no one else but me.

This is not to hide these stories from the world or you, the reader, but I hold them close because they were so life-altering and personally profound; these last ceremonies are just for me now, for my heart, soul, and being. I respect the culture that brought Ayahuasca to the world and will always hold it in the highest regard. Of you, the reader, I ask you to be okay with this because one day if you feel the call to sit with her, I don't want my stories to muddle your experience, I want you to go in with an open mind.

If you do have the honor to be in her presence with the Mistro's, be grateful, hold those moments close, be open, be honest, be willing, and most important, be ready to work. The ceremonies are just the beginning my friends, the work comes after. But if you protect the seed and light they place upon you, you can grow, blossom, and become the most powerful version of yourself. I have and will continue to heal because of those around me I have been given the gift of sitting with Ayahuasca and I will never ever stop thanking them for this.

You all know who you are, you gave me the chance to be myself. The good, the bad, the dark, and ugly—and now, the light. The patience so many around me have shown me is more than most get in a lifetime, I love and thank you all, my husband, my family, and my pack.

IYKYK.

TWENTY-SEVEN

Closure

August 2021

Months after my first time sitting with the medicine in 2021, the world flipped on its head. What came next was desperately hard to watch for a lot of people, little alone be a part of. The world watched as Afghanistan fell into the hands of the Taliban once again after twenty years of war. Griff and his team stepped up like many, and he reached out and asked for some help.

It was time to move some people, it was time to jump back into Afghanistan.

Just a little different than last time.

My phone rings. It's Griff.

"Hey, so I've got a pack of nine Canadian visa holders; I need you to try and move them."

"Hey, um I have no routes or ways of moving them."

"Try, because if you can't, then they stay in Afghanistan, they will be hunted down. Two are VIP."

"Alright, I guess were moving them then."

Who was I to say no—not after what my friend's kindness had done for me.

The fall of Afghanistan in August 2021 was heartbreaking, to say the least; it was earth-shattering for a lot of people. The Afghan people had spent twenty years with the presence of foreign soldiers keeping the fighting at bay. And now, almost overnight, it was all crumbling. So many Afghans grew up working with and for the NATO forces. So many people were feeling a lot of mixed emotions over why and how the pullout was being done, leaving so many people behind with no real plan on how to get equipment or people out. The clock was running out, fast. This was going to be bad; most just never thought it could go as bad as it did—until Afghan began to fall.

Canada was doing little to get people out—less than little, actually. My government held a snap election for prime minister and the media was specifically instructed to not cover or speak about what was happening. This came directly from a reporter who called me the week of the pullout asking "to interview Canadian veterans because they must be angry." The reporter's words, not mine. Gaslighting much?

You're fucking right we were angry, and we, like everyone else, had a right to be! Shocker, our prime minister didn't want the world to know he was abandoning Canadian visa holders in the country, with no one to contact or help. We were watching as Americans and Brits flew in to support. Canada sent a small, small amount of people. Less than a hundred Canadian soldiers were ready to go, but we were getting word they were being stood down. Visas and IRCC (Immigration, Refugees and Citizenship Canada) paperwork and other documents weren't being authenticated, we had no one to call to even confirm people's documents. That would be an issue, a huge issue. Little did I know at the time, that would be the least of my worries.

I received a few phone numbers on the encrypted messaging app Signal, and I began communicating with the family I was going to try to help. I knew little about them, just a few names. One of the women in the group had a husband who was studying in New York, and he and I began communicating right away.

Let me be clear: This is not the world I was in when I served in Afghanistan. Nowhere near it. I was a gunner, a grunt, not someone who understood, or even understands now, how to do things like moving humans around. But I was willing, like so many, to help because part of me was still hurt from the way I left that country, and I didn't want to see it fall this way. Not after so many soldiers lost their lives on that soil fighting the good fight.

August 23, 2021

Like many, Brass & Unity started by getting on social media and posting videos. I didn't know where else to start, so that felt like a good place to start:

"HEY HUMANS! We need some help, we need to get in contact with someone on the ground please dm (direct message) us."

To my surprise, we got hit right away with message after message. People wanted to help! That was a relief, but now we had to go through all our contacts to see how far we could get up the chain to someone on the ground making decisions.

If you know anything about the military, things take time.

But we didn't have time. We had one week to get these people on one of the only flights out of the country before they—like so many who had families who served in their government, police, or worked with a NATO country during the war—would be hunted down.

The Taliban were going door to door looking for people on a list:

Who was an interpreter?
Who helped Americans fight the Taliban?
Who promoted women's rights, education, and freedoms the Western world had?

They were looking for anyone who opposed them.

This family had a target on them.

The first female VIP was Shabnam, the women's rights commissioner for the Afghanistan Independent Human Rights Commission (AIHRC).

The second female VIP was Walwala, the senior gender advisor and director of women's cricket in Afghanistan.

Shit. How the hell am I going to pull this off?

Enayat, Walwala's husband, who was in New York while the country fell, and I began talking, with me realizing how terrified he must be with his family stuck in a country that was collapsing all around them. We got to work getting the families' passports, IRCC paperwork, visas, photos, and anything else we would need to make this go.

We had about one week before the last fight was scheduled to leave, and that meant we had to get documents authenticated by someone.

Once again, it became apparent that the new podcast I had started the year before would come into play here, the same way it had with ayahuasca.

About six months before Afghanistan fell, I was introduced to an absolute power couple for the podcast. Mutual friend Geriant Jones, veteran, author, and podcaster, asked me if I would be interested in interviewing Dean Stott.

Dean was a British special operator who had just broken a Guinness World Record on a road bike. I was eager to discuss the ride with him, so we agreed to have him on. Very quickly after speaking with him, I realized how incredible and powerful his wife was, and that's when I had Alana Stott on the show. Alana, being a powerhouse all on her own—close protection officer, founder of Wolfraven Omnimedia, and author.

At the time of the interviews, I had no clue how meeting those two would ultimately be one of the key reasons that we could even attempt moving these people out of Afghanistan.

While waiting for my contacts to come through, I knew my best chance would be to ask Alana for help. I knew there was no way her and Dean's company would just be sitting idly by and watching. So, I made the call and, sure enough, she was doing exactly what I thought she would be. On the phone day and night getting things done while running her company and managing two kiddos—just being the overall powerhouse I already knew she was.

She asked me what paperwork we had, and to send everything we knew about the Afghan family over. That week, I put aside my responsibilities at the office and at home to just be by my phone, available 24/7. The eleven-hour-and-thirty-minute time difference to Kabul was a big swing, so it left little time for sleep.

That meant that Walwala's family, who was waiting on the other end of the call, didn't sleep much either. And to make matters worse, their three-year-old boy just got beaten by the Taliban at the gates of the Kabul airport. Things were getting heated, and we needed to get this child some type of medical attention.

Alana came back with some questions about ages and visas, told me to hold tight, and that her people would be verifying as soon as they could. In the meantime, we needed to keep the family safe. We had them move to a safer location the next day and wait until we could clear the documents.

At this point, I wasn't even sure how or who we could get to grab this family. It was becoming apparent that getting people through the main gate just wasn't going to happen.

We received a contact through an Instagram message:

"Hey, I know you don't know me but I have a buddy who is inside the airport and he said he might be willing to help."

I messaged this guy back and gave him my number.

Thirty seconds later I get a call.

"Hey, I know this is crazy but my name is B****** and I have a friend who can help, I'm going to give you his cell. Contact him as soon as possible but listen...this is a long shot and he can't promise anything, but he said he would try."

I thought to myself, *Fuck it what do we have to lose?*

I needed someone on the ground, and fast. I added the contact and texted him on Signal.

"Hey I got your number from B****** he said you might be able to help me."

"Hey, ya how many?"

"8pack and one child who needs medical asap."

"How bad's the kid?"

"Bad enough."

"Alright, no promises, send the documents you've got."

"Sent."

At this point, we ran into a problem—the Americans were coming to get the VIP but couldn't take the family. I asked them please over and over "do not separate!" If they did, there was a chance the family wouldn't be high enough value to get the rest of them grabbed, but the family had no choice: Shabnam had to go. We were down to eight people. At this point, the Canadian contact we had just bailed on us, and the rest of the Canadians were leaving, so I now had to rely completely on the British and Americans. Sounds familiar doesn't it? Story of my life. But I trusted Alana and Dean and had no choice but to trust this American stranger on the other end of Signal.

We needed to move the family again to get somewhere safe; we were getting reports of Taliban going door to door looking for Western sympathizers. I wasn't willing to let them be sitting ducks, so Enayat and I went back and forth, and I finally got the family to agree to move once more.

Another random message on Signal: "Hey, I hear you need some help."

"Ya, we've got guys looking for this family, im not sure who you've been talking to but there a bunch of people trying to get them on a evac list."

"Instagram man, just trying to get to anyone who can help."

"Alright sit tight, here's this number ********** give this to them. Tell them when that number calls them, to pick up the phone. DO NOT MISS THAT CALL."

"Got it. What's your name? And who are you with?"

"Americans, thats all you need to know."

"Sounds good to me."

The next day, August 26, a suicide bomber blows himself up at the Abbey Gate of the Kabul airport, killing nearly two hundred people, including thirteen U.S. Service members.

Things just got a lot more complicated, and fast. The family was become more worried about going anywhere near the gate now. Understandably so, but we had to get them inside those walls one way or another.

By now, the Americans had taken the high-value member of the family, and the others were up to me and the people helping us. The little one was getting worse, and we needed to move quickly.

We got the call from Alana, she said we were good to go, the paperwork was authentic, and gave me what I needed to pass along to the people on the ground. Without Alana giving me the go, we were dead in the water.

Relief!

We had what we needed, now we needed someone to either go outside their command or find a contractor in the country who would make the attempt and get these eight people into the airport.

I got a call from the first Signal messenger: "Look we aren't sure we could guarantee getting these people into the airport, but we can try going by ground."

"What does that look like?"

"On one of the buses, drive them to the border and fly them from Pakistan."

"How would that work?"

"Move at night, bribe the guys at the checkpoint and get them through."

"And if they can't get them through?"

"...we can try, we can't promise."

I got on the phone and called the family, and they didn't like that option. But I was running out of options; I didn't know if I would be able to get them on a plane at all, and this might work.

I asked them again: "Are you sure you don't want to try this way? Once we turn it down, I can't get this option back."

"We are sure, Kelsi, please keep trying another way."

I reached out to the second person, the "American" on Signal and said:

"Look, I know you don't know me, but I really don't have another option for them here, can you try."

"Look Kelsi, ill see what I can do but right now after the gate went sideways and if we do this it's going to go fast, and we won't have a lot of time or many chances to get this done."

"That's fine, just try please."

"Ill get back to you soon"

(Following are transcribed voice memos and text messages of our movements from the week Afghanistan fell, with photos and screen shots.)

August 27

I was standing on my back deck screaming into my phone while my son and husband watched from inside the house. I must have looked crazy and the neighbors probably thought I lost my mind. It was go time; this was the moment we were waiting for.

The American messaged and said they were emptying busloads of people and then their guys were going out to get them.

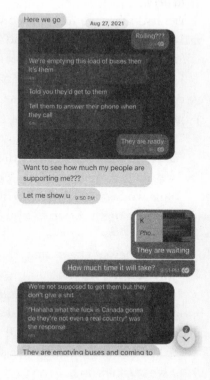

"We're not supposed to get them but they don't give a shit."

"Hahahah what the fuck is Canada gonna do, they're not even a real country."

I was slightly offended but didn't have time to care, these guys were willing to do what my government wasn't. Help—never leave anyone behind.

Call comes in: "We've got two chances, if they miss the windows, I can't help any further, okay? Tell them to stay by their phones and wait for your call."

"Got it."

I got on the phone with the family and said: "Listen this is what's going to happen, I need everyone to do exactly what I say as soon as I say it. We have two windows of time we can try and get you into the airport, but we can't question everything I'm asking you to do, just work with me here."

"I am here and waiting." Walwala says.

I messaged Enayat and said it was go time, and that I needed a photo of the family in the clothes they were wearing, and needed it fast.

Americans message back: "Im need you to get your family to this side street near the airport, I'm going to give you coordinates now, tell them to hurry up and send me a photo of them in the clothes they have on today."

I got on the phone with the family and said: "I'm going to give you a location and I need you to get in a car and get there ASAP! This is our time, this is the green light we've been waiting for."

Americans: "Tell them to wave a red scarf when they get to the location."

"Got it."

Message to the family: "What color scarf do you have on?"

The family responds: "We have different color scarfs, my sister is wearing a red color."

Message to the family: "When you get to the location, send me a photo of what you see."

Family: "Here, there is barb wire in the middle of the road."

Americans: "Send the photo of them, I need my guy to know who he's looking for."

"On it."

Message to the family: "I need the photo!!"

Family: "Here!"

Message to Americans: "Here, they've got a red scarf."

"RGR." (Roger.)

Message to the family: "Are you there yet? Wave the scarf, wave the scarf!"

Family responds: "Im sorry but it is impossible, the police man is not letting me, he told me to leave the area or I will shoot on you."

Message to the family: "No, no, no, get out of the car and go stand in the middle of the road, I need you to stand in the middle of the road and wave it above your head."

Family: "We are waving the red scarf, we are in the middle of the road, no one is responding. There's a sounds of firing also. Where should we go?! Where should we go?!"

Message to the family: "Walk further west, and get on service road. It's the side road going west. Stay behind the crowd, don't get into."

Family: "Kelsi we just left the area because they are shooting! And firing! And doing some bombing."

Message to the family: "DON'T LEAVE THE AREA! Go west and get on the service road. Go west now. Time to be brave and get on the service road now."

Message to Americans: "Whats that smoke?! Family is panicking and running."

Americans: "I can confirm that's us, tell them to stay there and walk toward the smoke, I repeat that smoke is us."

At this point, Enayat was getting upset, worrying and messaging. I kept asking him to keep communications clear, I needed the family's full attention.

Message to the family: "That is the Americans! Walk toward the smoke, walk toward the smoke, it is not tear gas, you're fine! Now is the time to be brave, WALK TOWARD THE SMOKE AND KEEP MOVING! That smoke was for you!!"

Americans: "I'm about to send my buddy out to grab them, if he gets hit. It's on you."

"Great, thanks."

Americans: "No problem, tell them to look for the big man with a big beard in a t shirt."

Message to the family: "WALK TOWARD THE SMOKE! There is a big American with a big beard in a t shirt looking for you. GO NOW!"

Family: "Kelsi I went to the point with the red scarf, but the police man said I cannot wave the scarf and he looked at me and said don't wave it, don't wave it. And then he came and we went away."

Message to the family: "Please stop arguing and listen, I need you to walk toward the smoke and wave the scarf, fuck the police officer I need you to walk and wave the scarf!"

Family: "I cannot its impossible, the policeman told me to leave the area otherwise I will shoot on you."

Message to the family: "Walk towards the smoke, if you don't your life is over you do not get it! Walk toward the fucking smoke, please listen! That smoke is for you, do not walk away again please! Hold the scarf, don't wave it then, just hold it. Youre going to see a giant fucking American man in a t shirt with a huge beard, once you see him start waving the scarf. We dont have time for you to question this decision, please JUST WALK TOWARD THE SMOKE. STAY IN THE SMOKE, THEY ARE COMING! Just stay there! Stay there!"

Americans: "Alright, hes coming out now, have them ready."

Message to the family: "Here they come!!! HOLD THE RED SCARF UP NOW!! Hold it up! Here they come, the Americans are coming! Stay right in place, please stay still!"

Americans: "Jackpot."

I dropped to my knees and screamed: "YES!!!!"

My son walked to the back door that leads to the back deck and says, "Mommy! Did we win?!"

I replied, "Yes baby, we won!"

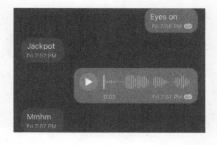

Yes baby, we won. That moment will be burnt in my mind forever. When my son grows up and asks me about that day, I will stand up with pride, shoulders back, and explain what we did and exactly how we did it, all because so many risked themselves for this family. Because that day, we did win, and a family was safe from the Taliban once and for all.

Message to the Americans: "THANK YOU, photo?"

Americans: "Tell them to take one, ive got more people to get."

"RGR."

Americans: "Right after your family, got another one."

"Well done man, I owe you a drink."

"No stress, just glad to help."

Message to the family: "I'm so sorry I had to yell, I just had to get you to move. I'm so sorry."

Family: "It is not a problem, I can understand, if you didn't yell, I couldn't pass the road, thank you."

7 more please

Very time sensitive

This if for when they come

I have the photo of the baby 6:44 AM

Do you know a Canadian in airport? 6:45 AM

They are all gone

I need the photos Enayat

Priority now 6:45 AM

them? 10:34 PM

Stand by

Don't bug them I need their comes

Comms

Hold ok 10:34 PM

Everything ok? 10:34 PM

Yes please stop

I need comms 10:35 PM

Bombs and tire gases are firing

Nargis

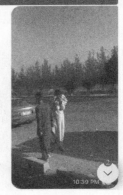
10:39 PM

0:04

How long !! I need to no?!

10mkn???

GO GO GO 10:12 PM

12 kilometers 10:12 PM

What color scarf will see wave 10:12 PM

One second 10:13 PM

Need photo

YOU CAN DO THIS

I believe in you!!! Breathe we can get them now 10:14 PM

10:17 PM

0:04 10:18 PM

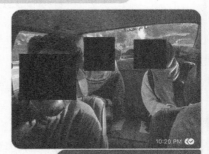
10:20 PM

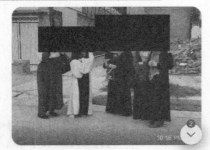
10:16 PM

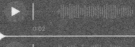
0:02

0:03

0:04

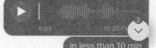
0:03 10:20 PM

In less than 10 min

They are happy their eyes tell the story of hope 11:49 PM

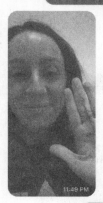

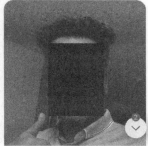

Ok 10:15 PM

Moving fast 10:15 PM

Faster 10:16 PM

Get me my people

NO SHOT

Oops 😅

That was to him

▶ |‖‖‖‖‖‖‖‖‖‖‖‖‖‖‖‖‖‖
0:07   10:17 PM

Ink 10:17 PM

TELL WALWALA TO DROP ME A LIVE PIN 10:17 PM

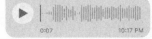

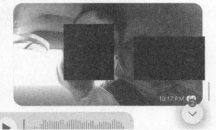

They will 2:37 AM

Move when u can safely 2:38 AM

Ok noted 2:44 AM

☏ K called you · Aug 27, 2021 5:01 AM
☏ K called you · Aug 27, 2021 6:34 AM

Call Back

Quickly for the photos very time sensitive 6:35 AM

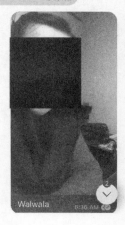

Walwala 6:36 AM

Praise be to god 🙏 Aug 27, 2021

He doesn't know how this change means to him

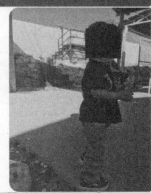

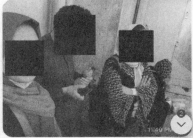

11:49 PM

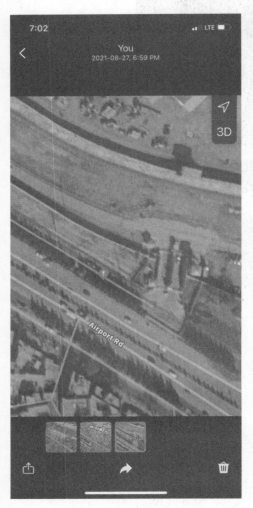

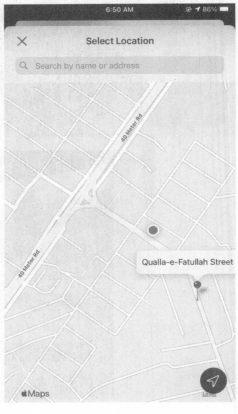

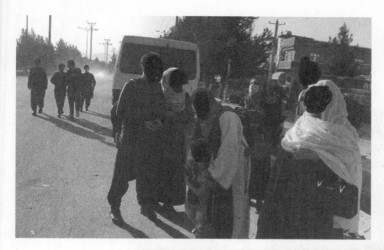

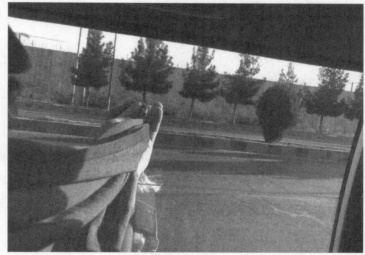

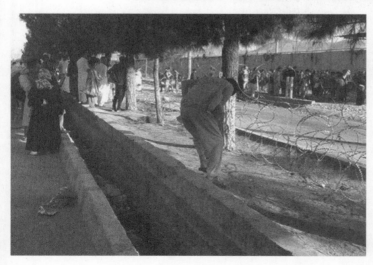

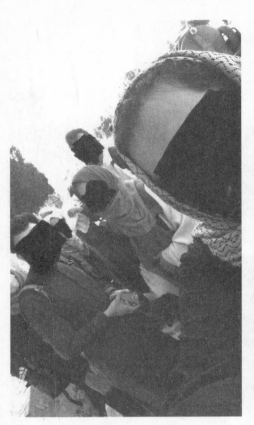
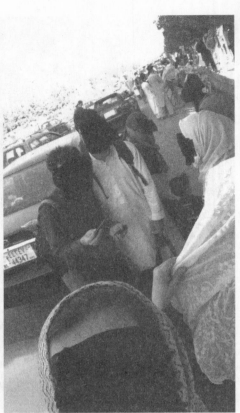
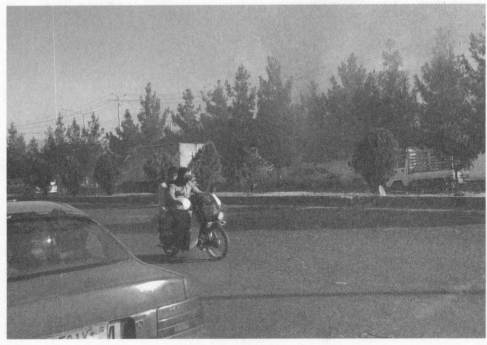

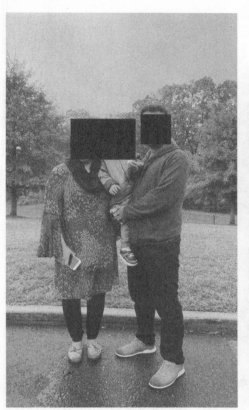
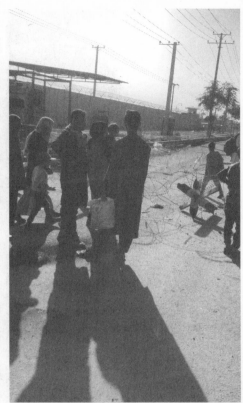
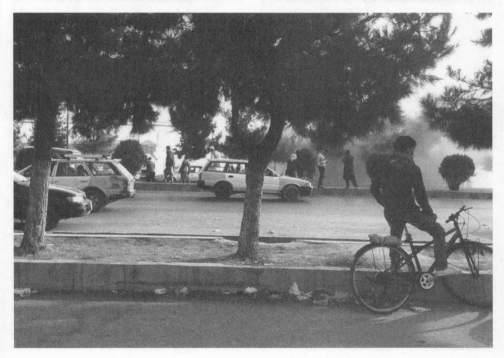

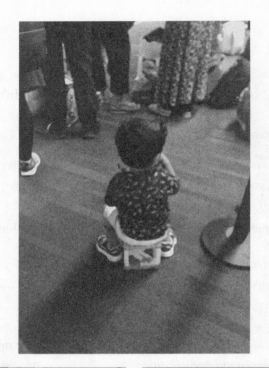

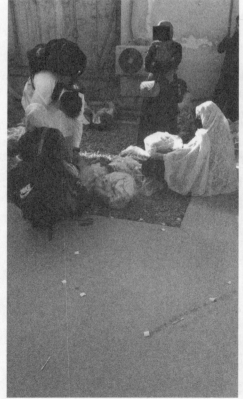

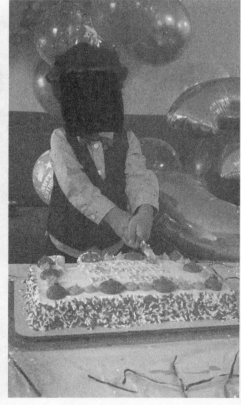

A few days went by, and I knew the family was on a flight out of the country, but I wasn't sure to where. Frankly, it didn't matter; they were gone, away from the fear and oppression of the Taliban, but I won't lie, I was excited to find out where they would land.

I received a message from the family a week later: "Hello Kelsi, hope you are fine. We are in Italy and awaiting a flight. They say it will take many days but we will see."

Message to the family: "But you are all safe and that's all that matters."

Family: "Yeah, fortunately, and I really thank you for your support and the struggles."

Message to the family: "It was no struggle for me."

Family: "You will always be in our hearts. You will see how your contribution helped a family find a bright future, once again, thank you for all you did and are doing."

Message to the family: "I'm here and will make sure you make it over. It might take some time, but I'm still here. Please send photos once you arrive and reach out if you need anything. I'm following your movements on my end and making sure you get what you need."

Another few weeks passed and I received another message: "Hello Kelsi, hope you are fine. We are in New Jersey. We arrive yesterday. My mother and sisters are in contact with Canadian embassy and they will move to a hotel today or maybe tomorrow. I am leaving for New York in three hours. Other people will spend three months or more at the camp, as I have a child it becomes difficult to spend more days at the camp, he is sick and doesn't eat anything here, so I decided to skip the process and move to New York. This is because of your support."

Message to the family: "That's amazing! Please send photos when you are all settled, I'm so happy."

We began sharing photos back and forth of our families. They sent along the video of the little boy reuniting with his father. It was all the most beautiful experience.

To this day, I keep in contact with this family and the Americans who moved this family, saved their lives, and gave them a new beginning.

To those Americans: You know who you are. I will always be in your debt, A.

* * *

As I sit here, almost one year to the day after the Afghanistan pullout, I can't help but look back and reflect on that time in my life. We all go through different journeys in life, and each one is meant to teach us something. Moving the family also helped me heal.

I didn't realize while I was doing it, but I was finally closing the Afghanistan chapter in my life. I was letting go of what happened there and how I left, I was moving forward in my healing by helping others.

People were left behind, and I will never find that acceptable, but helping one family was enough for me to move forward. You can't always fix everything in the world, but you can fix and work on yourself if you're open to it. Open to doing the hard work, and hard work it is.

Life since the military has been full of ups and downs, but I can say I'm on a different path now, one that allows me to help and heal at the same time. There is a lot of work to still do on myself, but I am no longer broken, I'm just cracked.

And cracks...well, they can be fixed.

We all experience difficult times in our life, but how you choose to look at those difficult times will determine how or if you grow. Regardless of how your trauma happened, trauma is trauma, and it affects everyone differently.

Try and remember wise words by Christine Caine, "when you're in a dark place you think you've been buried, but you've actually been planted."

Trust me, this is just the beginning.

About the Veteran Crisis

Often the systems that are put into place to help veterans are overloaded and inefficient. Here are just some organizations that are making a difference.

(Apologies if I missed anyone; so many are doing the hard work and I am grateful for them each and every day.)

Heroic Hearts Project
Defenders of Freedom
The Boot Campaign
Veterans Exploring Treatment Solutions (VETS)
All Secure Foundation
Warrior Angels Foundation
Canadian Legacy Project
Homes For Heroes Foundation
Honour House
True Patriot Love (TPL)
Valour Place
VETS Canada
Wounded Warriors Canada

Building Homes for Heroes
Special Operations Association of America (SOAA)
Kirstie Ennis Foundation
NINE LINE Foundation
Overwatch Project
Rescue 22 Foundation
Green Beret Foundation
Coast x Coast Foundation
REORG Charity
C4 Foundation
FitOPS Foundation
One More Wave
The Pat Tillman Foundation
The Special Operations Warrior Foundation
The Veterans Project
Help for Heroes
The Royal British Legion
Soldiers, Sailors, Airmen and Families Association (SSAFA)
Survive to Thrive

If you're struggling, one of these organizations will help you, or connect you with someone who can.

If you need immediate assistance, call the Veteran Crisis Hotline at **1-800-273-8255** and **press 1**.

Send a text to **838255** to receive confidential support twenty-four hours a day, seven days a week, 365 days a year. This service is for veterans and their loved ones.

Coping Tips

Neither operating a business nor writing this book would be possible if I didn't have some control of my PTS symptoms. As you can see throughout the book, through the ever-present voice of PTS, it doesn't go away. I live with the symptoms of PTS all of the time, and without coping strategies, it can easily take over. Remember that PTS is an injury, and it has to be treated like an injury.

Even with my therapies and support systems, writing about the darkest parts of my life has been triggering and painful. In the pages that follow, I share the things that worked for me throughout my healing journey, as well as things that didn't work for me but might work for you.

Remember, if you are in crisis, call the Veteran Crisis Hotline: **1-800-273-8255** and **press 1**. Send a text to **838255**.

Psychedelics

Look into them if you feel like you have hit a plateau, if you feel the calling to look at an alternative way of healing. They are not a cure all, but they have allowed me to see a different way of healing. There are organizations out there that can help you decide if this type of medicine is right for you. Speak with your doctor before, especially if you are on any medications or have a history of mental illness in the family. Always consult a professional before taking anything. Know what you're getting yourself into, because psychedelics are not a magic pill. They require support, integration, and a safe setting with people who specialize in facilitating the plant medicine that is best for you.

Art Therapy

Art therapy was a lifesaver for me, and through Brass & Unity, it has grown into something fulfilling that allows me to help a lot of people—exactly what I set out to do when I joined the military in the first place.

Jewelry-making worked for me, and maybe it will work for you. Maybe it won't. The point is to find something that quiets the PTS voice for a while. If you keep your mind busy, there's a chance PTS will shut up, and that's what happened for me. I strung beads onto string, and that simple process kept my brain too busy for flashbacks.

Check out your local community center and find out if there are art classes you can sign up for. Sometimes they're free, sometimes you can get a military discount. You may find a place that offers a program they can slide you into.

Talk Therapy

I continue to see Dr. Passey consistently, every single week, and he holds me accountable for my shit. If you have access to a psychiatrist, please explore that option. If you do not have access to a psychiatrist, find yourself a fellow vet and reach out to him or her to talk.

Movement and Touch

I was a highly competitive athlete my entire life, so exercise has always been a priority for me. I believe that when you take care of your body, you're also helping the health of your brain. You can see a difference in my symptoms when I am not on top of my fitness game. Being active is a major part of my treatment in order to keep me level. Find some way to be active. Try running or go for a walk, join a gym. Just move your body. For best results, be consistent.

Massage therapy is very healing for the body. Check if you have coverage, and if you do, take advantage of it.

Yoga and meditation are also helpful for the mind and body. If you don't have access to yoga classes, check out YouTube. If you don't have access to YouTube, hit up the library and find a book about how to get started.

Nutrition

Do your best to eat healthy, drink plenty of water, and sleep eight hours a night. I'm not a doctor and do not claim to be, but I know that eating healthy will help with your treatment process. At least it has for me.

Cannabis

Now that cannabis is legal in Canada, it obviously is easier for us Canadian vets to access it. Cannabis helps me cope. When I started using cannabis as recommended by my doctor, I saw improvements in my general mood, sleep, and overall quality of life. It helps to reduce my triggers and has made me feel so much better. If you are in Canada, ask your doctor if cannabis might work for you. If you're in a state in the U.S. where it's legal, do the same.

Journaling

Journaling is something that doesn't always work for me, but it might for you. A doctor recommended that if I wake up from a nightmare, I should write it down, and that might make it easier to get back to sleep. I continue to try and add this into my daily life. I use journaling now to work on my mental wellness, help me keep the positivity moving. Gratitude journals can be found at any book store and can be a great start.

Significant Others

Having a significant other that understood trauma and could be there for me is something I was blessed with. Not everyone is so lucky, but finding someone you can trust to lean on will help. There are many programs available for couples, since PTS can have a big effect on a marriage. It's important to communicate if you're struggling and attempt to work through it together.

A combination of some of these things may work for you, but I know what won't work for you: suicide.

When you live with PTS, sometimes you have to be okay with not always being okay. I hope one day anyone struggling will recover from war or trauma, but sometimes people succumb to their injuries. I think everyone has the potential to get better and to embrace the new version of whatever that is.

* * *

If you think someone is hurting or suffering from PTS or other traumas, please reach out and don't let that person suffer in silence.

If you are an actively enlisted soldier, a veteran, a police officer, or a first responder, I hope you are able to draw a bit of strength, knowing that a barely five-foot-tall kid who went to war and came back broken was able to claw her way out of the darkness and begin to heal.

Please don't give in to the awful voice of PTSD. I want to see you in Valhalla when it is our time to go. Not a minute before. Let's make the twenty-two suicides per day of the present a thing of our past. If you need immediate assistance, call the Veteran Crisis Hotline at **1-800-273-8255** and **press 1**. Send a text to **838255**.

USA: The 988 Suicide & Crisis Lifeline is a national network of local crisis centers that provides free and confidential emotional support to people in suicidal crisis or emotional distress 24 hours a day, 7 days a week in the United States.

Acknowledgments

To the people whom I've met and worked with on this project over time: I'm grateful to you for your patience, kindness, empathy, and understanding. I am aware that, over the past four years, this hasn't been an easy process of which to be a part of, and those who have stuck it out have helped me to achieve a dream of becoming an author and helping my community. I'll never stop holding space for you in my heart. I hope you all know who you are.

To Neal and Ruve McDonough: You'll never fully understand the love I feel for you and your family. Your big, beautiful family has welcomed me with open arms from the moment we met at our first Fire Career Rep 24-hour row-a-thon. You've continued to move mountains for me, and our next chapter together will be bigger and brighter. I thank you for taking a chance on me the way you both have.

James: You came to me with an idea for a charity event, a way to help others; and because of that, I was able to meet Neal and Ruve. Thank you, my friend, I promise to never forget this.

Tali, you stood by with patience and kindness and helped me walk through the last four years of this process. I am grateful to you for this.

My parents and family, this goes without saying. I love you and thank you for the patience and grace you've given me throughout this journey to heal.

To the soldiers I served alongside, those of you I keep in contact with—Canadian, American, British, and Australian: I love you deeply, I'll never forget anything you've ever done for me. You all know who you are, some of you are mentioned in this book and others have had your name changed to protect your identity. Thank you guys so, so much.

Dr. Greg Passey, there are not enough words or pages in this world to thank you enough for the man you are, and more importantly, the doctor you are. Your integrity as a doctor is unlike anything I've ever seen or heard of. You save lives daily. You deal with the Department of Veterans Affairs' BS like a champion and have kept me moving and growing and answered the phone no matter the time. You, sir, are one of the greatest gifts the military has ever seen, and to any person who has the chance to be your patient. Thank you now and thank you later, because I know you're my doctor for life. I owe you, sir.

Jack, my son. One day you'll be old enough to read this and talk to me about it; I promise to be open and honest with you about everything and answer any questions you have. I love you, my son, you are the greatest gift and the BEST thing I've ever done in my lifetime. Thank you for choosing me as your mother; I only hope I can make you proud one day. I love you.

To my unwavering, strong, brilliant husband. I owe this all to you and your compassion, your patience, and your belief that I could do anything I wanted in this world. You really have made me believe I can achieve it all, and now I plan to because of you. Your strength is the reason I still stand today, I love you forever and always, Roo.